1776: Medicine and War

Doctors and the Battle for America

Ronald S. Gibbs

ISBN-13: 979-8-9967705-0-2
Imprint: Independently published

Cover design by Judith Lippe and Howard Bomze
Printed in United States of America

Dedication

In memory of Jane Holtz Gibbs

Table of Contents

1776: Medicine and Revolution

ILLUSTRATIONS

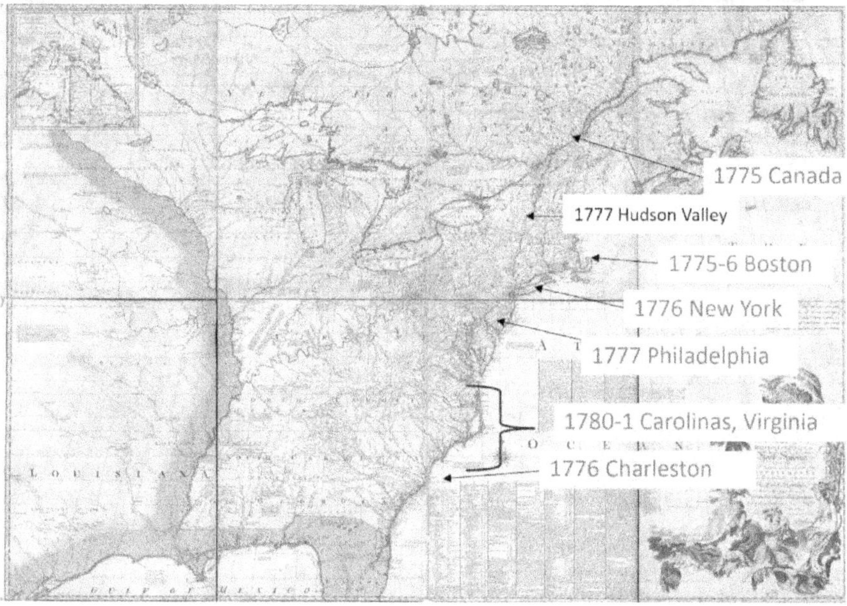

MAP OF THE AMERICAN REVOLUTION. SUPERIMPOSED ON THIS MAP OF THE BRITISH COLONIES IN NORTH AMERICA (BY JEFFREYS AND FADEN, LONDON, 1775) ARE DATES OF THE MAJOR ACTIONS OF THE WAR. THE FIGHTING BEGAN AROUND BOSTON IN 1775 AMIDST A SMALLPOX EPIDEMIC AND ENDED IN YORKTOWN, VIRGINIA IN 1781 AMIDST A MALARIA OUTBREAK. MAP, COURTESY OF LIBRARY OF CONGRESS GEOGRAPHY AND MAP DIVISION.

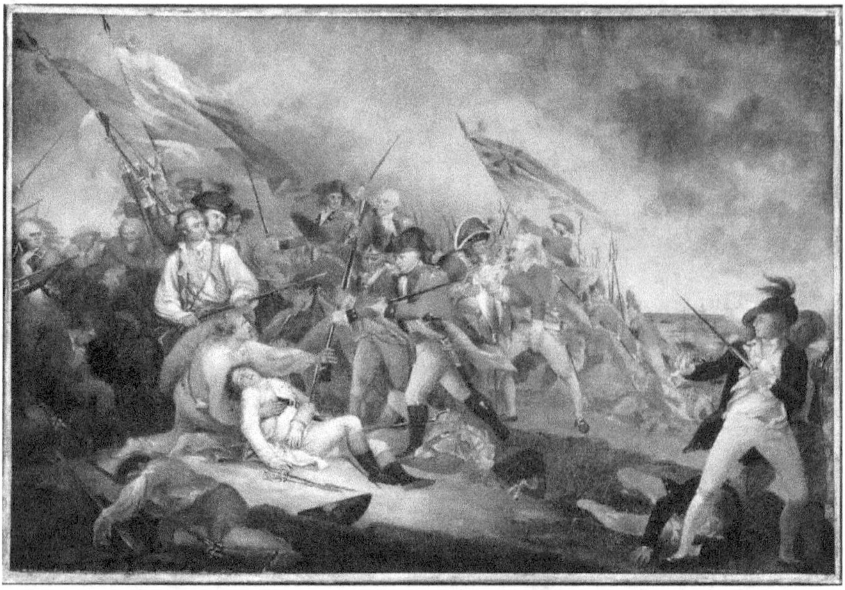

"THE DEATH OF GENERAL WARREN AT THE BATTLE OF BUNKER'S HILL, JUNE 17, 1775" BY JOHN TRUMBALL, 1786. JOSEPH WARREN WAS A NOTED BOSTON PHYSICIAN, PATRIOT LEADER, AND MAJOR GENERAL IN THE MASSACHUSETTS MILITIA. TRUMBALL'S PAINTING DEPICTS HIS HEROIC DEATH AT THE END OF THE BATTLE. IMAGE, COURTESY OF YALE ART GALLERY.

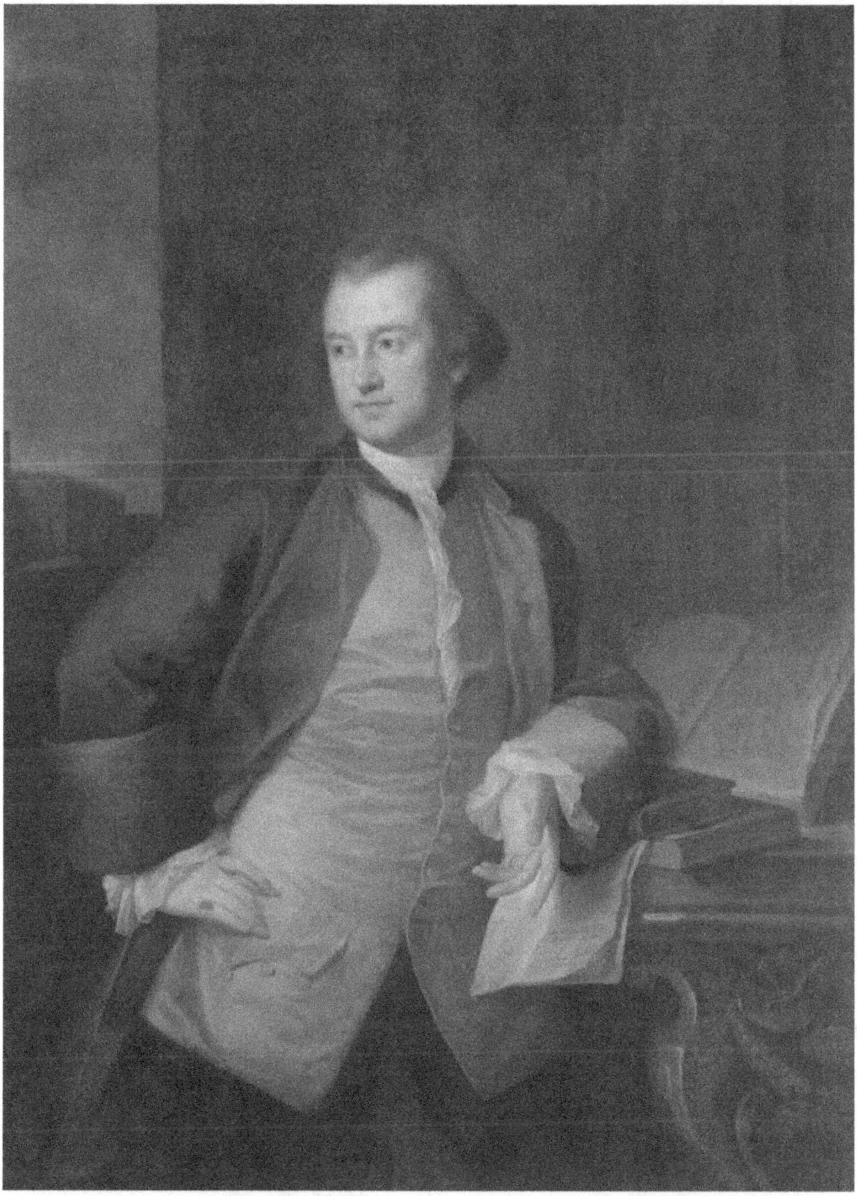

JOHN MORGAN, BY ANGELICA KAUFFMAN IN 1764. MORGAN WAS ONE OF AMERICA'S MOST DISTINGUISHED PHYSICIANS. HE CO-FOUNDED THE FIRST MEDICAL SCHOOL IN THE COLONIES IN 1765 AND SERVED AS THE SECOND DIRECTOR-GENERAL OF THE CONTINENTAL ARMY MEDICAL DEPARTMENT. HOWEVER, BECAUSE OF INFIGHTING AND ADMINISTRATIVE DIFFICULTIES, CONGRESS FIRED HIM AFTER JUST FIFTEEN MONTHS. PORTRAIT, COURTESY OF NATIONAL PORTRAIT GALLERY.

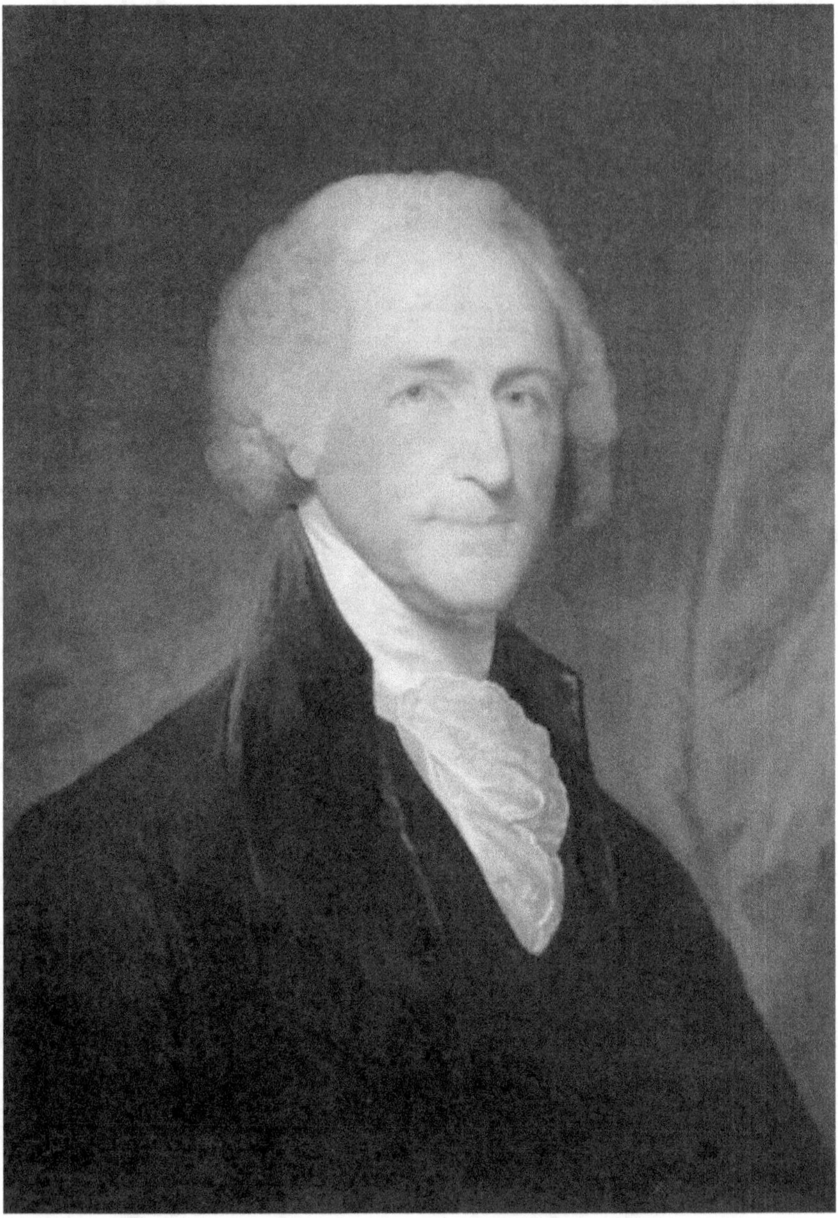

WILLIAM SHIPPEN BY CHARLES WILSON PEALE, DATE UNKNOWN. ALSO ONE OF THE MOST PROMINENT PHYSICIANS IN THE COUNTRY, SHIPPEN CO-FOUNDED THE FIRST MEDICAL SCHOOL (WITH MORGAN). HE SUCCEEDED MORGAN AS DIRECTOR-GENERAL OF THE MEDICAL DEPARTMENT, BUT HE TOO HAD A ROCKY TIME, WINDING UP BEING COURT-MARTIALED FOR MISCONDUCT AND IMPROPRIETIES. HE WAS ACQUITTED BUT SOON RESIGNED. PORTRAIT, COURTESY OF UNIVERSITY OF PENNSYLVANIA.

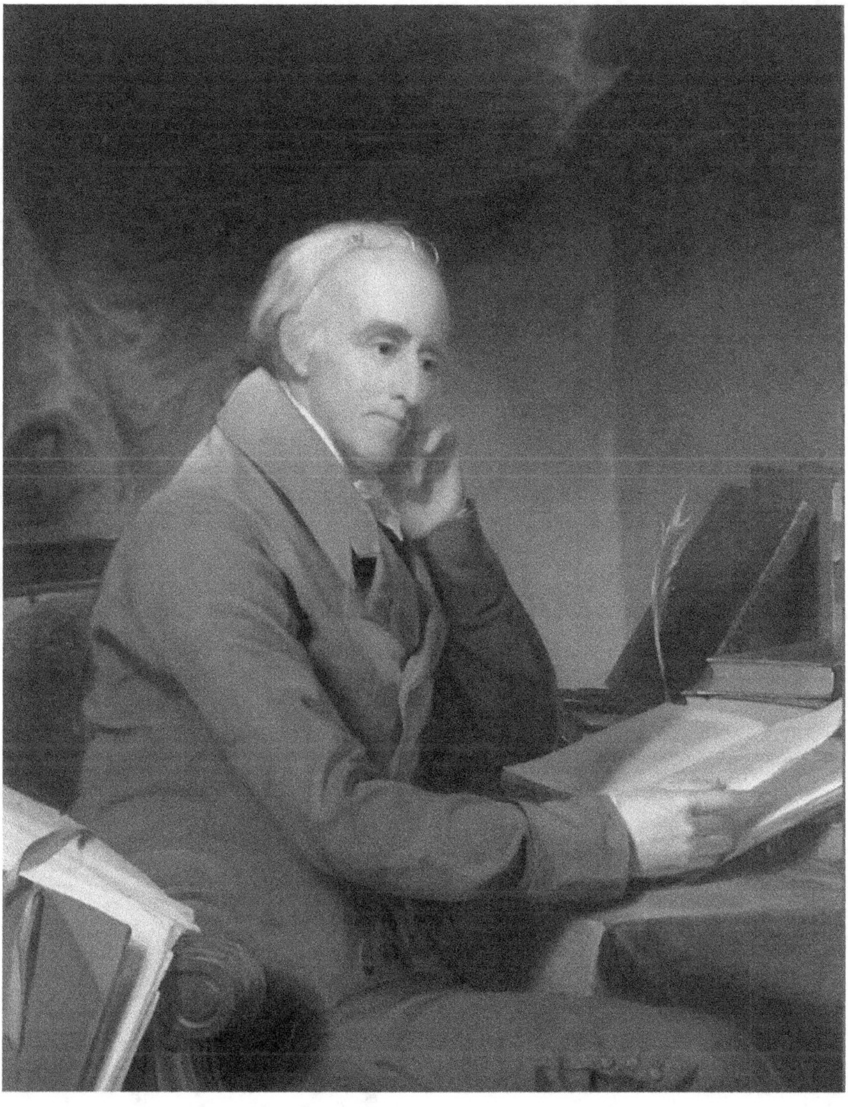

BENJAMIN RUSH BY THOMAS SULLY, 1812. ONE OF THE MOST REMARKABLE AMERICAN PHYSICIANS OF THE ERA, BENJAMIN RUSH WAS A MEMBER OF CONGRESS, A SIGNER OF THE DECLARATION OF INDEPENDENCE, AND SURGEON GENERAL OF THE MIDDLE COLONIES DURING THE WAR. HIS PAMPHLET ON PRESERVING THE HEALTH OF SOLDIERS, WRITTEN IN 1777, GUIDED PREVENTATIVE CARE IN THE MILITARY THROUGH THE AMERICAN CIVIL WAR. RUSH CHAMPIONED HUMANE CARE OF THE MENTALLY ILL AND IS CALLED "THE FATHER OF AMERICAN PSYCHIATRY." PORTRAIT, COURTESY OF NATIONAL PORTRAIT GALLERY.

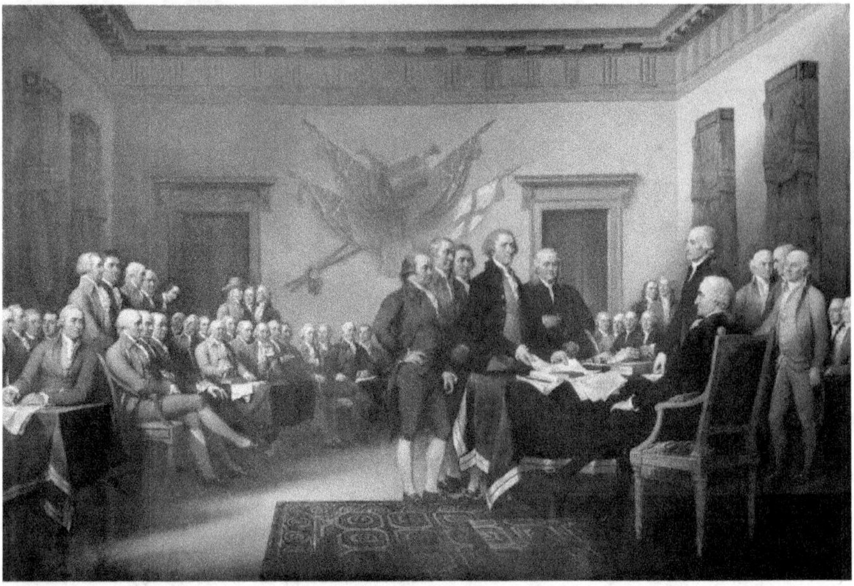

"THE DECLARATION OF INDEPENDENCE, JULY 4, 1776," BY JOHN TRUMBALL, 1786. IN THIS ICONIC PAINTING, TRUMBALL SHOWS 47 FIGURES BUT NOT ALL THE 56 SIGNERS. THREE OF THE FIVE PHYSICIAN-SIGNERS ARE INCLUDED IN THE PERIPHERY. FROM LEFT, JOSIAH BARTLETT IS THIRD, BENJAMIN RUSH IS NINETEENTH, AND OLIVER WOLCOTT, FORTY-FIRST. DRS. LYMAN HALL AND MATTHEW THORTON WERE NOT INCLUDED. PAINTING, COURTESY OF YALE ART GALLERY.

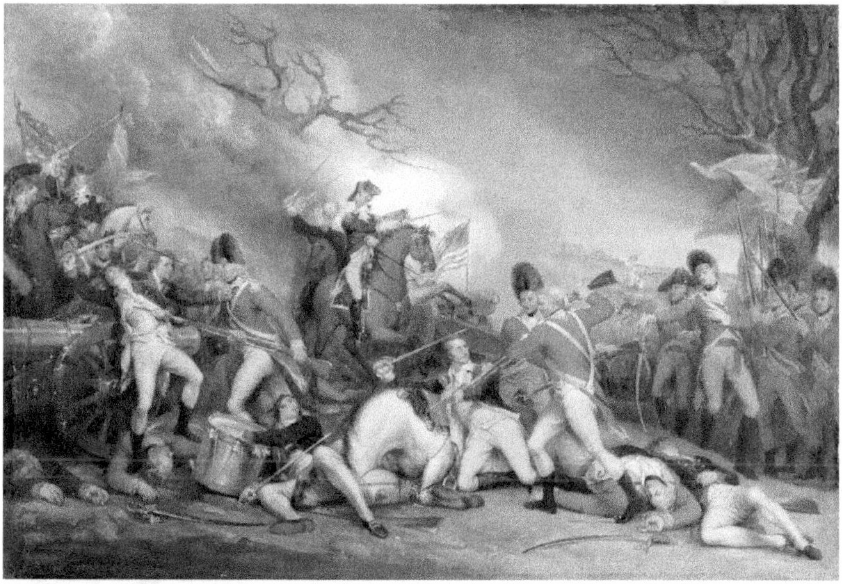

"THE DEATH OF GENERAL MERCER AT THE BATTLE OF PRINCETON, JANUARY 3, 1777" PAINTED BY JOHN TRUMBULL TEN YEARS AFTER THE BATTLE, DEPICTS THE WOUNDING OF MERCER, AN AMERICAN GENERAL AND DOCTOR. THE PAINTING WAS TRUMBULL'S FIRST DEPICTION OF AN AMERICAN WAR VICTORY. IMAGE COURTESY YALE UNIVERSITY ART GALLERY.

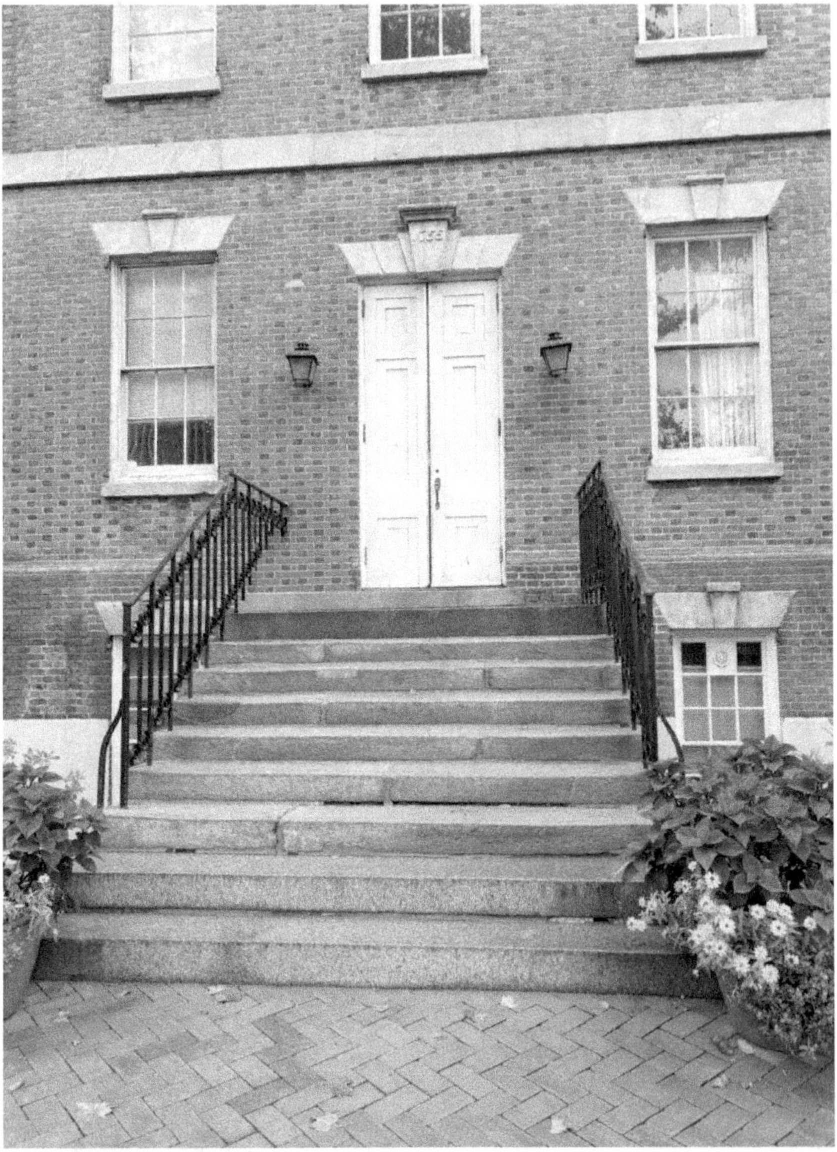

PENNSYLVANIA HOSPITAL, THE NATION'S FIRST, WAS FOUNDED BY BENJAMIN FRANKLIN AND DR. THOMAS BOND IN 1755 WITH A MISSION OF "CARING FOR THE SICK, POOR, AND INSANE WHO WERE WANDERING THE STREETS OF PHILADELPHIA." THE FIRST PATIENTS WERE ADMITTED IN DECEMBER 1756. THE MEN'S WARD WAS ON THE FIRST FLOOR, THE WOMEN'S WARD ON THE SECOND FLOOR, AND CELLS FOR THE INSANE IN THE BASEMENT. THE MODERN HOSPITAL STANDS ON THE SAME CAMPUS IN HISTORIC PHILADELPHIA. PHOTO BY AUTHOR.

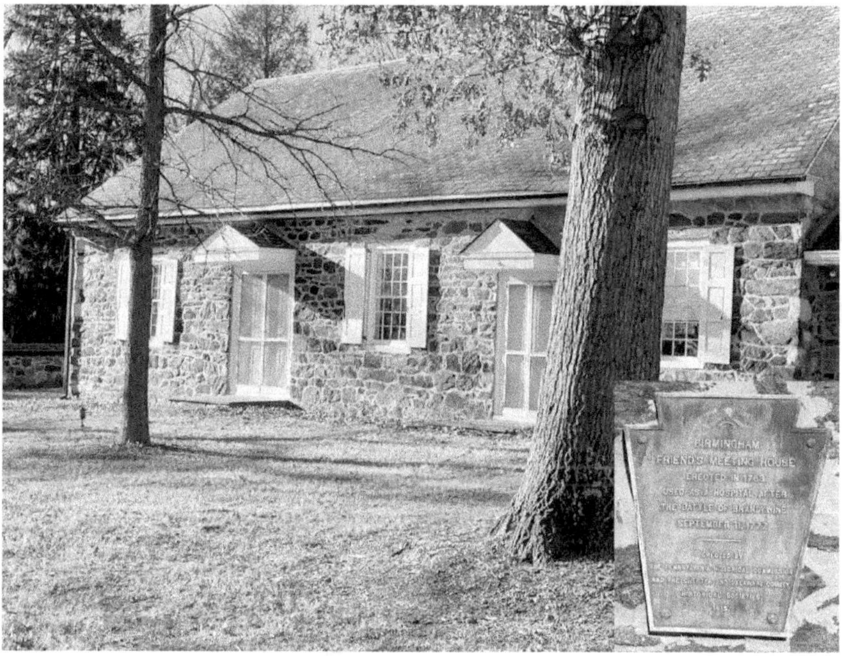

The Birmingham Friend's Meeting House, erected in 1763. Located near Chadd's Ford, Pennsylvania, the stone meetinghouse was used as a hospital after the Battle of the Brandywine on September 11, 1777. Inset historical marker. Photo by author.

PREFACE

During the American Revolutionary War, General George Washington's army faced two enemies. One was mighty, well-armed, disciplined, and fresh from victories in Europe and North America. These were the land and sea forces of King George the Third of Great Britain. The other enemy was still invisible in the Eighteenth Century but much more deadly. These were the germs that took advantage of the conditions of war to cause disease and pestilence. Doctors of the day saw the ravages of these microscopic enemies but had no idea of their cause, only the basic ideas of their contagion, and little concept of effective treatment. The result was devastating. Diseases claimed three fourths of all the deaths among the men in Washington's army. The best estimates are that among the 230,000 who served at one time or another in the Continental Army and among another 145,000 who served in the militia, 7,000 were killed in action, but about 20,000 died of disease.[1]

Before the Revolutionary War, North America was considered a relatively healthy corner of the British world, especially in comparison to crowded, polluted London. The thirteen colonies, spreading 1300 miles from New Hampshire to Georgia, were mostly wilderness, populated sparsely by about three million persons, a sixth of whom were enslaved. The largest city was Philadelphia, Pennsylvania with a population of just 30,000 compared to London's of 750,000. Over ninety percent of the people in the colonies lived on farms or in small towns and villages, and nearly all resided within a few dozen miles of the Atlantic coast. Transportation was by foot, horseback, coach, wagon, carriage, or boat. On a good day, one might travel twenty-five to thirty miles. It would take ten to fourteen punishing days for a rider to travel the 300 miles from Boston to Philadelphia. Roads were dirt, and in rainy or snowy seasons, they became impassable. Few American colonists ever traveled very far from home or ever visited a large city. Most led isolated lives having contact with small numbers of people.

Yet, even in North America, disease was an everyday part of life in the Eighteenth Century. Life expectancy at birth was just thirty-two years. Child mortality (death between birth and age five years) was tragically about thirty percent though once a child survived the first five years, life expectancy rose to age forty-seven for men. If a man made it to age fifty, he could expect to survive until his seventies.[2] (Gifford does not specify here, but these data most likely pertain to free white men). The chief cause of death was infection arising from the unseen micro-organisms, but other common causes were trauma and bleeding. For women, life span on average was even less than for men because of death from complications of childbirth. The death rate from pregnancy was about one in 100 (1-1.5%). As one modern historian summed up the time of the revolution, "Disease was a constant fear embedded on the American psyche."[3]

Medical practice was stuck in ancient concepts, not very different from the Greek and Roman times. It was an era of treatment with bleedings, leeches, and laxatives, all well-intended but harmful. The physician's armamentarium was limited, and there were few effective drugs. The great advances of medicine were still seventy-five to one hundred years in the future when systematic study of anatomy, biochemistry, micro-biology, and pathology led to scientifically based medical and surgical treatments.

When the Revolutionary War broke out, conditions got even worse. Not just for the soldiers but also for civilians, there was great uprooting. Huge masses of men and women were all crowded together in military encampments or overflowing in cities. Around New York City in the fall of 1776, the combined strength of the British and American forces was over 50,000, equivalent to the populations of North America's two largest cities (Philadelphia and New York) combined. Fearing the consequences of the British occupation of New York in 1776 or Philadelphia in 1777, many patriot families boarded up their homes and left.

The citizen-soldiers of the Continental Army who had previously led isolated lives became exposed to new and lethal diseases. Camps were unsanitary, allowing pests and pestilence to proliferate. Summer in North America is hot and humid, but the heavy uniforms of both opposing armies were of wool or linen, with little opportunity for washing. During the harsh winters, the American Army encamped at strategic positions to keep an eye on the British, but suffered in crowded, crude, poorly heated log huts. And in all seasons, diet was poor with regular shortages of fresh vegetables and meat. Wartime conditions welcomed disruption, disease and death.

In paintings of American Revolutionary battles, there are heroic depictions of men wielding muskets, swords, and bayonets or firing field cannons with great blasts of ball and clouds of smoke. It's easy to conclude that most deaths in wartime would be from battlefield injuries, but in fact it was just the reverse. As mentioned earlier, only twenty five percent of the deaths were from battlefield wounds. The comparatively low number of deaths from battle were mainly attributable to the military technology and strategy of the times. During the American Revolution, there were few pitched battles in each campaign. In 1775, there were only two main battles. In the 1776 campaign, there were a total of seven. And in the critical year of 1777, there were just six large battles. What's more, weapons were slow firing and had short ranges. Accordingly, battle casualties were relatively low. At Lexington and Concord in 1775, for example, American killed and wounded numbered 89, and even at Bunker Hill, the number of patriot casualties was just over 400. The next year, at the Battle of Long Island (Brooklyn), with 10,000 American soldiers involved, the number of American killed and wounded is estimated at only 200. It was the convergence of the conditions of war, the pre-scientific state of medical care, and the state of military technology that made disease, not battle, the most prolific killer of the army.

The other seventy five percent of deaths among the soldiers occurred from disease exacerbated by the crowded, undernourished, under-clothed, under-housed and often cold and wet conditions of military life coupled with the physical demands of marching and fighting. Too often the soldiers were under-served by the pre-scientific state of medical arts.

The purpose of this book is to tell the story of medicine during the Revolutionary War from a unique perspective. The first section views the war primarily through the eyes and words of real-life doctors and nurses. It encompasses how they faced not only devastating diseases and maiming wounds but also despair and even their own frailty when some took deathly ill themselves. The second section deals with how physicians contributed to the revolution—as warriors and statesmen—and how they helped build the nation through innovation, courage, and heroism. Chapter One, in recounting how the American army tried to make Canada the fourteenth state of the union, encapsulates issues of strategy and command structures that would continue throughout the war. Chapter Two explores George Washington's personal experience with smallpox and how that influenced not only the Continental Army's policy but also quite likely the outcome of the war. Chapters Three through Nine examine the roles of various Revolutionary War medical practitioners in fields ranging from surgery to nursing, as some tried to instill hygienic standards into medical practice and upgrade hospital care and others indulged personal arrogance and inflexibility leading to disarray in the Medical Department at the expense of caring for the soldiers. Chapter Ten zooms into the most common diseases and the art of treating them, and the preparation and education available to the physicians of the era. The subsequent chapter looks at the implications of the state of medicine for some of the notable patients. Starting with Chapter

Twelve, the book recounts true tales of medical practitioners and their unique roles in shaping the values of the new country. A surprising number of physicians gave up their medical practices and became high ranking military officers. Signers of the Declaration of Independence were disproportionately pulled from the ranks of physicians, as were public servants in positions of power.

I started formally researching this topic in Philadelphia and London while I was a third-year medical student in 1968 as recipient of a Logan Clendening Traveling Fellowship in the History of Medicine. Over the decades, I kept two shoe boxes full of index cards with detailed references and notes. Those shoe boxes survived eight family moves, and I was able to recover data collected in 1968 from original sources in London. Overall, my references span 300 years.

I wanted to make the story readable but capture the flavor of the primary sources. These quotes enrich the story and give personal perspectives from those experiencing the times. To keep the flavor of Eighteenth-Century prose, I have maintained these quotes with their convoluted sentences and punctuation and spelling.

I have included occasional references to currency. In the new United States, the dollar was used as opposed to the pound in Britain. For reference, an American captain's pay was about forty dollars per month. A cow cost about ten to twenty dollars.

In researching the era of 250 years ago, I encountered numerous gaps. To fill in the story, I tried to stay as true to the times as I could in creating scenarios, for example, of how a surgeon would likely have performed an operation.

Based on a lifetime of reading and studying medicine, I have aimed to put knowledge and practice of the Revolutionary War era in the context of modern practice. To keep the story of

Eighteenth-Century medicine flowing, I placed the great medical developments of the Nineteenth and Twentieth Centuries into informative footnotes. In addition, for readers with a great thirst for more extensive detail about diseases and surgery, I have added Appendix B.

This book is a work of non-fiction, written by a physician but aimed at a general audience. I trust it will serve as an engaging tour of Revolutionary War times highlighting important medical personalities, their collaborations and conflicts, and the treatments they practiced, sometimes highly effective and often curious to Twenty-First Century readers. As such, it will serve as a companion to my historical novels which relate the history of the early years of the Revolutionary War as seen through the eyes of its protagonist, the appealing widower and capable physician Alexander Grant. These novels, *The Long Shot, The Secret History of 1776* and *The Rogue's Plot, The Untold Story of 1777,* allude to the challenges faced by physicians and their military and civilian patients. Now, amidst the 250th anniversary of American Independence, *1776, Medicine and War* tells an intriguing and under-appreciated story of our country's founding and its medical quandaries, some of which persist to the present.

---

[1] American Revolution Facts, website.

[2] Gifford, 73.

[3] Abrams.

PART ONE:

DOCTORS BATTLE AGAINST DISEASE

CHAPTER ONE

DR. ISAAC SENTER ENCOUNTERS SMALLPOX, 1775-1776

The heroic invasion of Canada

Convinced that the Canadians would welcome the opportunity to become the fourteenth colony and join the revolution against the British, in late 1775 the Continental Congress authorized an expedition to invade Canada. Under the command of Colonel Benedict Arnold, who at this point was a bold and effective officer, an American army of 1100 men set out to capture Quebec City. Arnold's small army sailed from Cambridge, Massachusetts in mid-September, landed on the Maine coast, and then headed into the Northern wilderness toward Quebec, over two hundred miles away. Owing to their start late in the season, they were about to encounter epic hardship from severe weather and ravaging disease. Among these men was Dr. Isaac Senter, surgeon, just twenty-two years of age.

Dr. Senter was born in 1753 in Londonderry, New Hampshire and moved to Rhode Island as a youngster.[1] Like nearly all the doctors in the North American colonies, he did not attend a medical school but instead carried out a medical apprenticeship.[2] Afterwards, Dr. Senter opened his practice in Cranston, Rhode Island. Just after the Revolutionary War broke out in April 1775, he joined the Rhode Island militia which then became part of the American forces surrounding the British Army in Boston.[3]

When Colonel Arnold's invasion force to Canada was organized that summer, Senter was appointed its surgeon despite his relative lack of experience. It seems likely that no senior surgeon was willing and available.

Hardship in the northern wilderness

Young Dr. Senter had his hands full at the start.[4] We know this because he kept a detailed medical journal. By September 27th, as the troops made their way north by boat and on foot, "several of our army were much troubled with the dysentery, diarrhea, & c".[5] Senter must have expected to encounter dysentery because it was one of the most common and severe diseases among soldiers in the field. The men likely developed dysentery from the combined effects of poor sanitation, crowding, spoiled food, and contaminated water. Senter recorded that many casks of food had burst, souring the bread and spoiling the peas. Barrels of salt beef were also damaged, rendering the meat "not only unwholesome, but very unpalatable".[6] Nearly a month later, the troops were still making painstakingly slow advancement northward and were continually troubled by dysentery. On October 24th, as the troops were exposed to "a direful howling wilderness" and an early season snowfall six inches deep, Senter wrote, "Several of our men were excessively exhausted with the diarrhea".[7]

Despair began to set in. Senter wrote, "Several of the men ... were ready to give up any thoughts of ever arriving at the desired haven. Hunger and fatigue had so much ascendancy over many of the poor fellows ... that some of them were left in the river, nor were heard of afterwards."[8]

The invasion force nevertheless made it to the St. Lawrence River and sailed across on November 13th. Encamped outside Quebec City on November 21st, Senter found "our army had been tolerably healthy since our arrival over the river, but ... more than usually cold weather, & c. produced ... some severe "peripneumias" (pneumonias),"anginas, (chest pains)& c."[9]

On December 5th, half a mile from Quebec's St. Roques' Gate, Senter commandeered "an elegant building situate[d] upon St. Charles River," as his general hospital. It had "a chapel, nunnery, and hospital all under one roof." He wrote, "The number of sick were not very considerable at this time, however, they soon grew more numerous."[10]

In the harsh winter climate, respiratory infections including "pleurisy [and] peripneumonia" became "very prevalent in the army",[11] and on Sunday, December 17th, the first cases of smallpox broke out. Five men required admission to the hospital. Smallpox was feared as it was one of the most virulent and contagious of all diseases with virtually all exposed persons becoming infected.[12]

Although Dr. Senter does not say whether he had seen smallpox earlier in his career, he probably did during the large outbreak in and around Boston that had begun in November 1774 and continued through early 1776. He was in the American camp encircling Boston from May to September 1775. Senter may have also seen sporadic cases in Rhode Island during his apprenticeship or practice. Even if he had not, he would have studied smallpox during his apprenticeship and would have known its characteristic findings.

From his education and experience, Dr. Senter would almost certainly have known that smallpox began with chills, severe headache, lower back pain, and vomiting. Doctors then did not yet have clinical thermometers, but Dr. Senter would have learned that fever was typically high in smallpox cases. He would not have known that it was caused by a germ nor that it had an incubation period of nine to fifteen days. An Eighteenth-Century doctor might have had difficulty making the early diagnosis of smallpox because its initial symptoms overlapped with other illnesses, but suspicion of smallpox was heightened if there were an outbreak in the camp or if the soldier had a direct exposure to another infected person. When there was suspicion of smallpox, even before the onset of the classic rash, the doctor would likely quarantine the patient who was already contagious.

Young surgeon Senter would have confirmed the diagnosis of smallpox with the appearance of the disease's characteristic findings: small, raised skin bumps (called papules), usually on the fourth day, progressing to fluid-filled blisters (called vesicles) with a central dimple, or "umbilication" for its similarity to a belly-button on the fifth or sixth day, and developing into small. grayish-yellow pus-filled pockets (called pustules) by the eighth day. In severe cases, the rash covered the whole body. In fatal cases, by the tenth or eleventh day, the pulse weakened, and the patient became delirious. Complications in severe cases included pneumonia, hemorrhage, persistent vomiting, seizures, and coma.

Dr. Senter does not describe his treatment of smallpox while in the wilderness, other than to say that some patients were sent back to the Maine coastal towns, nor does he state what medications he had available. It is likely that he set out with a reasonably complete medical chest and would have been able to apply bleedings, emetics to induce vomiting, and cathartics to evacuate the bowels. For pain, he would have used an early opium derivative such as gum opium or laudanum.

So common was smallpox in the Eighteenth Century that everyday men and women in Colonial American would have also known about it, often from a personal or family experience because it was so contagious that it spread through trade and other means even to remote locations. One estimate is that smallpox killed over 100,000 people in North America during the revolution as it "swept across the continent and ravaged cities, armies, villages, plantations, and Native Nations".[13] In Boston, with a population of about 10,000, there were epidemics in 1722 when nearly 6,000 caught the disease and later in 1731 when 3600 had it from natural causes. Smallpox cut across all classes. In 1736, Benjamin Franklin's young son Francis died of smallpox, and a few years later, one of Paul Revere' s children became severely ill but survived. In the epidemic of 1752, half of Boston's population became infected with smallpox.[14] Occurring with damning regularity, smallpox outbreaks infected Boston residents again in 1764 and once more in 1774. Other large cities such as Charleston in 1738 had their own epidemics. The death rate in these epidemics hovered around fifteen percent to seventeen percent of those afflicted.

The disastrous attack on Quebec

With the Canadians showing no desire to join the rebellion, the American command decided to storm the walled city. Arnold's troops were joined by General Richard Montgomery's men who had captured Montreal a few weeks earlier. The joint attack was carried out under cover of darkness amidst a blizzard on the night of December 31st. Senter described the storm as "tremendous," with "snow not less than six feet deep".[15] The attack was a disaster, easily repulsed by the British regulars and the Quebecois with heavy American losses. Within an hour of its start, "the wounded came tumbling in [to the hospital so] that the grand ward was directly filled." At daylight, Dr. Senter found out that his commander had been shot. "Colonel Arnold was brought in ... wounded in the leg with a piece of musket ball."[16] Recording that the ball lodged in Arnold's calf muscle "at the rise of the tendon Achilles," Senter "easily discovered and extracted it." A week later, Senter noted that Arnold had "so far recovered of his wound" and after several more weeks went on to full recovery. Several other American officers were wounded, and later that morning Senter learned that General Montgomery had been killed by British cannon fire.

Knowing they could not take the city by force, the Americans were obliged to lay siege to Quebec through the brutal Canadian winter. The American force was now about to be hit by a medical calamity that would dwarf the effects of dysentery, pneumonia, pleurisy, hunger, and fatigue. Epidemic smallpox was about to rain down on the army.

Epidemic smallpox

Cases of smallpox grew rapidly among the men, all crowded together and exposed to the subfreezing conditions. There was a prevention technique—called inoculation—but, despite being used in North America for over fifty years,[17] it remained controversial for use in the army for a variety of reasons. It was controversial because in all cases, illness followed. During this post-inoculation illness, the soldier was unfit for duty for up to two or three weeks when full recovery ensued in nearly all cases. However, in about one to three percent of inoculations, the case had a fatal result. Further, those inoculated could spread the disease and had to be routinely isolated. These downsides made inoculation unpopular among many soldiers and led to its prohibition by the army at the time. The upside of inoculation was that it provided complete, lifelong protection from the natural disease, but in the opinion of American medical officers such as American General John Thomas, himself a physician from Massachusetts, the downsides outweighed the advantages. The Continental Army, facing a much large enemy force, simply could not afford to have so many fighters out of commission while they recovered from inoculation. General Thomas ordered all inoculations to be stopped, and the Continental Congress concurred.

The Continental Congress was taking a gamble. Most American soldiers grew up in rural areas and had not had either the natural infection or inoculation. Many of them must have gladly accepted the orders against inoculation, but according to Senter, some, including "several officers",[18] feared getting natural smallpox so much that they resorted to inoculating themselves, even at the risk of severe punishment, including the penalty of death.[19] One technique used by the men was to "inoculate themselves by injecting pus under their fingernails."[20]

Because these self-inoculated soldiers could not quarantine themselves, they added considerably to the spread of smallpox.

By April, the American force besieging Quebec (the survivors of Arnold's and Montgomery's troops) numbered about 1400, but half of the men were sick with smallpox.[21] Congress was still committed to winning over Canada and sent reinforcements to Quebec. By early May, there were 7000 American soldiers outside the walled city, but 900 (thirteen percent) were sick, mostly with smallpox. When British reinforcements from England sailed up the St. Lawrence on May 6, 1776, the disease-battered American force gave up its siege of Quebec and retreated toward Montreal.[22]

General Thomas commanded Dr. Senter to "repair to Montreal and erect an hospital" as smallpox "was still very rife in the army"[23] General Thomas had never had the disease and had not been previously inoculated. In solidarity with his soldiers, he refused inoculation, thus signing "his own death warrant".[24] Smallpox was so widespread that even General Thomas "caught the natural smallpox, sickened ... and died".[25] General John Sullivan had to come north to assume command.

To meet the epidemic's cases in Montreal, Senter took over for his hospital "a fine capacious house belonging to the East India Company ... convenient for nigh six hundred [patients]." There, in apparent disregard of the deceased General Thomas's orders, he "generally inoculated a regiment." Senter wrote that the inoculations led to only mild disease as the regiment was "able to do garrison duty during the whole time".[26]

With the army's prospects "still gloomy" and with it "weakened by the small-pox, and in every movement against the enemy unsuccessful,"[27] a retreat was ordered from Montreal on June 9th. From there, the army straggled down Lake Champlain and Lake George back to New York. The invasion of Canada was a political, military and medical disaster. The objective was never obtainable due to Congress acting upon poor intelligence, and losses were terribly one-sided. American killed and wounded numbered about 60, but over 400 were captured. British and Canadian loses were only six dead and nineteen wounded.

In retrospect, Congress should have had better intelligence about Canadian allegiance. The generals should have had a more coherent strategy and a more realistic assessment of the hardships of a late fall campaign through the Northern wilderness, and both the commanders and Congress should have appreciated the devastating effect of dysentery, respiratory disease, and ultimately smallpox on the mission. Senter's experience with the heroism and suffering of American soldiers experiencing both good and bad leadership at various levels of command and the successes and limitations of medical treatment, encapsulates problems encountered throughout the war and serves to set the stage for understanding medical treatment in the army throughout the revolution. Senter bitterly concluded,

> It seemed upon reflection, a strange series of unaccountable misfortunes, the product of various causes, but from none more than the unpardonable neglect either in our commanders, in not giving Congress a true representation of the state of the army from time to time, or if so represented by them, the fault may be sought for in the non-attention of the latter. Thus ended an expedition of nine months' continuance, the ill success of which in any other cause would have induced us to have renounced the principles.[28]

---

[1] Dr. Isaac Senter Papers, website

[2] Apprenticeships were one to seven years long and were informal, unregulated training experiences under supervision by practicing doctors.

Notes, continued

There were no acknowledged criteria for becoming an apprentice, and some trained with a physician who was a relative. There was no standard for what the apprentice paid his mentor, but one fee was reported to be the large sum of one hundred dollars a year (according to Griesemer). By the nature of the relationship, the apprentice's knowledge and skills were limited to the those of his mentor. See more on apprenticeships in the Colonies in Chapter 3.

[3] By the time of the revolution, the militia already had a long history in British North America. Able bodied men were required to participate in these citizen-soldier units which were organized for the defense of their towns and colonies against Native Americans and the French. These units were often informal, made up of part time, non-professionals. On the other hand, the regular American army, called the Continental Army, was full time, professionally trained, and paid by Congress. The basic infantry unit of the Continental Army was a regiment, made up of about 600-800 men. Regular army officers often thought the militia forces were unreliable in battle, but militia units supplemented the regular army and played crucial roles in numerous battles including Bunker Hill. Although most militia units fought against the Crown forces, there were Loyalists who formed auxiliary units of the British Army.

[4] The Journal of Isaac Senter

[5] Senter Journal,15

[6] Ibid., 18

[7] Ibid., 25

[8] Ibid., 34

[9] Ibid., 45

[10] Ibid., 46

[11] Ibid., 48

[12] Smallpox is spread from person to person or by fomites (objects which can carry infectious materials such as clothing and bed linens). It generally smoldered and then became epidemic when conditions were ripe such as during crowding, especially acute during wartime. Smallpox is caused by a relatively large, DNA containing virus, called variola.

[13] Wehrman, 5, 16, 18, 47.

[14] Smallpox, Inoculation, and the Revolutionary War, website

[15] Senter Journal, 51

[16] Ibid., 52

[17] This inoculation process consisted of making a small incision on the arm and then placing infected material from a pustule into the wound.

[18] Senter Journal, 57.

Notes, continued

---

[19] Reiss, 94

[20] Ibid., 95

[21] Ibid., 95.

[22] Ibid, 95

[23] Senter Journal, 58-59

[24] Smallpox, Inoculation, and the Revolutionary War, website.

[25] Senter Journal, 58-59

[26] Ibid., 58-59

[27] Ibid, 58-59

[28] Ibid., 60

Chapter Two

General George Washington Confronts Smallpox Inoculation, 1775-1777

As a lad growing up on an isolated farm in rural Virginia, George Washington did not need to worry about smallpox. That was mainly a disease of the immense, far off European cities such as London with a population of 750,000. Smallpox also caused regular outbreaks in some of the larger, crowded North American towns such as Boston, Massachusetts or Charleston, South Carolina with populations of 10,000 each. Yet even these colonial epidemics mattered nil to those living on plantations and farms. With most of the citizenry leading relatively isolated lives and having contact with small numbers of people, outbreaks in North American cities remained localized. Young George Washington and his family at Mount Vernon felt safe from smallpox and had no need for inoculation. However, for the future commander in chief, all that soon changed through an act of family obligation.

The fateful voyage

Always industrious, nineteen-year-old George Washington spent the summer of 1751 in the profitable business of surveying and acquiring land in the Shenandoah Valley of western Virginia. He returned to Mount Vernon to find that his revered half-brother's health was deteriorating badly. Lawrence Washington had been suffering from tuberculosis and thought that a damp, cold Virginia winter would exacerbate his condition. The Caribbean island of Barbados was considered a haven for people with lung disease, and Lawrence, then forty-three years old, hoped that a few months in the tropical climate would prove salutary. Lawrence would need companionship on the long voyage but could not take his wife since she had a newborn to care for. George was the obvious person. With a sense of duty, he agreed to accompany Lawrence. For George, it meant "sacrifice of the chance of finding some new bargains in frontier lands, [but] family obligation came first... That was enough. Everything else could wait."[1]

The brothers sailed from Potomac, Virginia on September 28,1751 and arrived in the settlement of Bridgetown, Barbados about a month later. There, Dr. William Hilary, who had vast experience in lung diseases, examined Lawrence and provided an unexpectedly encouraging outlook. Dr. Hilary concluded that Lawrence's disease "was not so deeply seated that it could not be cured."[2] The brothers found suitable board and lodging though at an "outrageously high" price of £15 per month (about $6000 per month in today's US dollars). Settling into island life, George was "almost overwhelmed by the beauty of the tropical landscape"[3], and the views were matched by the hospitality of the island's dignitaries who were eager to meet the Virginians.

Two weeks after arriving, on the morning of November 17th, George Washington awoke with a chill and high fever. By nightfall, he developed a severe headache and back pains. The symptoms continued unabated over the next three days. On November 20th, tell-tale red spots broke out on his forehead near the hair roots. In just a few hours, the spots progressed to papules and then to pustules. It was certain that he had smallpox, probably from an exposure on shipboard or in Bridgetown. With his strong and youthful constitution, Washington battled the disease over the next eight days. By the 28th the fever resolved, and the scabs began to peel off. Although his course was a mild one, it left him with life-long facial pits. Washington won his battle over smallpox, which at the time claimed the lives of between fifteen and thirty percent of those afflicted with the natural disease. His physician released him from his care on December 12th.

After recovering, George enjoyed dinners with Lawrence and Bridgetown notables nearly every evening, but Lawrence was discouraged. He dearly missed his wife and newborn daughter, and Dr. Hilary's prognostication for Lawrence proved overly optimistic. At this time, George could be of little help to Lawrence and felt a pressing need to return to Mount Vernon. With Lawrence in agreement, George made a final farewell to his ailing brother and sailed north on December 21st, in good health himself. He landed at Yorktown, Virginia on January 28, 1752 and actively resumed his business affairs. Lawrence remained in Barbados for a few months and then sailed to Bermuda, but the ravages of tuberculosis continued unrelentingly. He died there eight months later in July 1752.[4]

George Washington's journey to the Caribbean showed the sense of duty that marked his entire life. It was the only time he ever left the colonies that would become the United States. His bout of smallpox proved fateful in his later leadership roles: It gave him life-long, complete immunity as well as sympathy for the thousands of his soldiers who would suffer and die from the disease.

General Washington appointed Commander in Chief

Twenty-three years later, in June 1775, the Continental Congress in Philadelphia appointed George Washington as Commander in Chief of the American forces, who were then surrounding the British Army in Boston. Washington looked the part of a commanding general. Tall, powerfully built, and honorable, he had been wearing his military uniform at the meetings of Congress. Congress also selected him because, as a Virginian, he gave regional balance to the forces who were then almost all New Englanders. Others were passed over. John Hancock thought he should have been selected even though he had no military service. Two former British officers, Charles Lee and Horatio Gates, had command experience in battle but were not selected as they were British born.

But Washington was not without his shortcomings. Although he was an officer in the French and Indian War, he served only in the Virginia militia, never commanded a unit larger than about 700 men, and as a colonial was denied rank in the regular British Army. Washington resented this snub his entire career. Washington's lack of command experience was going to become all too evident as the first campaigns unfolded.

General Washington and his entourage left Philadelphia and rode to Massachusetts, arriving in the American camp in early July 1775. There, he inherited medical and military troubles that had been brewing for some years. The situation resulted from the convergence of intense crowding in Boston, onset of a smallpox epidemic, and controversy over inoculation.

The smallpox epidemic in Boston, 1774-1776

British regulars had been stationed in Boston since 1768 to enforce Parliament's Townshend Acts. After the "Boston Tea Party" (December 1773), the Crown responded by sending thousands more British troops to garrison the city. Boston was packed with many new arrivals, fresh from the weeks' long voyage from the teeming cities of England.

In November 1774, five children of two British military families broke out with smallpox, and another case developed in a soldier of the 59th Regiment.[5] Not surprisingly, despite attempts to contain it, by January 1775 smallpox cases spread to outlying communities. In March, smallpox spiked again in Boston when ten new cases were reported to the town's selectmen (that is, city councilmen), but these were only the tip of the iceberg. The British Military Governor, General Thomas Gage, had kept it quiet, but there were thirty-eight more cases aboard his hospital ship tied up at the wharf. As noted by a modern historian, "Boston was facing its largest outbreak in over a decade"[6] just as the fighting was about to commence. The selectmen received notice that the British hospital ship was going to be moved from the wharf. At a subsequent emergency town meeting, they voted not to begin general inoculation but rather hoped to control smallpox by vigilance and isolation of cases.

The inoculation controversy

General inoculation was a response that had been used by Boston public officials for previous outbreaks, as in 1764, but it had to be weighed carefully in view of its risks and benefits. Inoculation had been used in Asia and Africa for centuries before it was introduced into Europe in 1721. Lady Mary Wortley Montagu, the wife of the British ambassador to Turkey, had her young son successfully inoculated in Constantinople before returning to England. Lady Montagu and her friend, the Princess of Wales, took up the cause and introduced inoculation into England. Inoculation made its way to North America by a different route. The Reverend Cotton Mather of Boston learned about inoculation from Onesimus, his enslaved African servant. When smallpox broke out in 1721, Mather advocated for inoculation among the city's physicians, but only one doctor, Zabdiel Boylston, was convinced. Boylston began inoculating actively, and his results were dramatic. He inoculated 242 patients, with only six deaths. These represented a death rate of 2.5%, compared to the 14.6% death rate from natural infection that year.[7] Newspapers in Philadelphia spread accounts of inoculation's successes in Boston, and the practice became widespread. Its relative safety and its effectiveness were demonstrated in several subsequent epidemics. In Boston's 1730 epidemic, only 3.0% of 400 inoculated died,[8] and in the 1752 epidemic, only 1.5% of over 2000 inoculated died. Smallpox inoculation also provided the benefit of complete, life-long protection from the disease.

Yet, as noted in Chapter One, inoculation remained controversial because all of those inoculated became ill for up to two or three weeks. Usually, the course was mild though debilitating, but in one to three percent of inoculations, the case had a fatal result. Officials also knew that inoculated persons were contagious and had to be isolated to prevent spread of the disease. The amount of time freshly inoculated soldiers would be unavailable for combat could result in a severe shortage of fighters.

Adding to the controversy, smallpox inoculation was accompanied by high fees, ranging from one to five pounds (a range of about $135 -$680 in 2026 value), medical opportunism, and even outright fraud. On occasion, the public reaction became violent, once leading to the burning of an inoculation hospital in Marblehead, just outside Boston.[9]

In the years leading to the American Revolution, the disadvantages of inoculation led to bans in several colonies. In the 1760s, the South Carolina General Assembly forbade inoculation despite a recent outbreak in Charleston. In Virginia, inoculation had been made a "penal offense," but the practice continued by "driving it to secrecy." Individuals "even inoculated one another, without attention to isolation, and so became the source of an epidemic of the natural disorder".[10] (As late as 1776, Connecticut still prohibited inoculation, and New York had recently forbidden the procedure.)[11]

Some civilians and soldiers objected due to the fear of death from inoculation, and others thought it was unnecessary, particularly if they lived in rural areas. Many soldiers, fighting in the cause of independence, thought the decision about inoculation should be an individual one, not commanded by a central officer. As with so many current issues in America, from defining citizenship to vaccination for Covid-19 and other diseases, similar controversies have existed in America since the initial struggles for the establishment of the United States.[12]

The beginning of Revolutionary War, 1775

After a decade of political struggle about colonial rights, taxes, and trade, the war broke out in Lexington and Concord, Massachusetts, with the "shot heard round the world". On that fateful day of April 19, 1775, the British sent 700 men to Lexington to arrest Sam Adams and John Hancock, resistance leaders whom we today call patriots. Alerted, Adams and Hancock had already escaped. British regiments and town militia faced each other on the town green. It is not known which side fired the first shot, but a skirmish ensued, resulting in several Americans dead or wounded. The British then marched an additional seven miles to Concord to destroy a cache of American weapons. When they arrived, they found preciously few colonial arms, exchanged fire with the local militia across Concord Bridge, and then began their march back to Boston, having achieved neither of their objectives. Now the countryside was alarmed, and thousands of New England militia assaulted the redcoat column by firing upon them from behind trees and rocks. The tactic gave the Americans a one-sided advantage. The total American dead and wounded amounted to about ninety men, but the British suffered 246 killed and wounded, about a third of the original number marching from Boston.

For the next two months, the British hunkered down in Boston, surrounded by thousands of militiamen. On June 17th, the British awoke to find that the Americans had fortified Breed's Hill (commonly mis-identified as its neighboring mound, Bunker Hill), and American cannons threatened them in the town. The British commander ordered an immediate attack to dislodge the militia from their earthen fortifications—into withering American musket fire. Only on their third attempt—when American ammunition ran out—were the British able to take the hilltop fortification, but at great cost. Owing to the tactics, this was a bloody battle. American casualties totaled over 400, but British amounted to over 1,000. The toll was so heavy, including all the

British commander's staff except the commander, that he subsequently avoided frontal attacks in almost every battle.

Before Washington arrived, the commanding officer was Brigadier General Artemus Ward of the Massachusetts militia. As a non-physician, Ward had already taken some actions to prevent smallpox from spreading in the growing and crowded American camp. He ordered the militia to treat all the captured British soldiers as potentially infected with smallpox and had the prisoners placed in a house guarded by militiamen who had had smallpox.[13] Brigadier Ward worried that he could not keep smallpox from the American camp just by isolating the British prisoners and established a nearby house in Brookline as a temporary smallpox hospital.

To treat the hundreds of Bunker Hill casualties, Ward and the Massachusetts Provincial Congress in late June set up several hospitals, certain to keep those wounded in battle separate from those with smallpox. General Ward placed a guard at the smallpox hospital to prevent anyone from entering except the doctors and those with the doctors' permission.[14]

General Washington in command

In early July 1775, the Continental Congress assumed control of the army replacing the Massachusetts Provincial Congress, and Washington arrived to take over from Artemus Ward. From July 1775 to March 1776, about 10,000 British troops and 6000 civilians were cooped up in Boston, surrounded by a much larger Continental Army. Conditions in the city were ripe for disease. Every bit of food (hardly any of it fresh), forage, and supplies had to be brought in by ship. Because of the lack of fresh provisions, scurvy became widespread.[15] In late September, British General Howe had "near one-third of the whole numbers" of troops either sick or wounded.[16] In November, he gave orders to inoculate his non-immune troops, and learning of that order, many civilians sought inoculation as well.[17] An estimated 2,000 British soldiers were ill with smallpox with the majority most likely having symptoms after inoculation[18] or exposure to others who had been recently inoculated.

Smallpox was feared in the Continental Army. In view of the cases of smallpox in Boston, inoculation of some American troops began as early as July 1775 despite general orders against it, and guards were posted at Boston Neck to prevent susceptible individuals from moving in or out of the town.[19] In December 1775, four British deserters told the American command of a heinous plot. The British commander General Howe, they reported, was planning on what today would be called "germ warfare." One of Washington's aides-de-camp wrote that "several persons are to be sent out of Boston ... that have been lately inoculated with the smallpox, with design, probably, to spread the infection in order to distress us as much as possible".[20] When some of the refugees sneaking out of Boston soon developed smallpox, Washington wrote to President of the Continental Congress John Hancock, that he "now must give Some Credit" to the veracity of the scheme. Washington was aware that the British soldiers were being inoculated as "a weapon of Defence they are using against us," but even then, he did not order general inoculation for the American Army.[21]

Historians have pondered whether British General Howe intentionally planned to spread smallpox as an act of Eighteenth-Century germ warfare or whether he was merely trying to make Boston less crowded. In 1763, the British did attempt to infect native Americans during Pontiac's Rebellion.[22] However, General Howe liked Americans, fought alongside them in the French and Indian War, and tried to negotiate an end to the war as late as summer 1776. It would have been out of character for Howe to have hatched a germ warfare plot in 1775 against fellow Englishmen, even those in arms against him. In a recent article, three medical historians conclude that the evidence was unclear, but "at the very least [British Commander] Howe enabled its spread".[23]

A stalemate developed over the winter of 1775-1776, but in March Washington took advantage of a British oversight. He fortified Dorchester Heights overlooking Boston from the south. From this position, American cannons once again threatened the British Army, which had no choice but to evacuate Boston. On March 17,1776, the British Army numbering around 10,000 plus thousands of Loyalist refugees sailed from Boston to Nova Scotia but fully intent on returning to their colonies to crush the rebellion.

As the British left, Washington was still suspicious that "the enemy with a malicious assiduity, have spread the infection of smallpox through all parts of the town".[24] Washington permitted only men who had previous smallpox to enter Boston.[25] In fact, cases of smallpox were "far lower than many expected." The Boston selectmen set up hospitals for the infected residents, and Washington wrote in his orders of March 20 that "Every possible precaution will be taken to destroy the Infection of Smallpox".[26] By early April, Washington was looking beyond Boston. He anticipated the full-scale return of the British to New York and began to march his army there.

The Battle for New York, 1776

Washington knew of the ravages of smallpox in the ongoing Canadian invasion in early 1776 (see Chapter One) and of the fear that soldiers and potential recruits had of contracting smallpox while in the army. Connecticut Governor Jonathan Trumball sent a letter to Washington on July 4, 1776 explaining that fear of the infection "operates strongly to prevent Soldiers from engaging in the Service" and that Connecticut battalions "fill up slowly".[27] In New York State, General Philip Schuyler raised identical concerns writing that potential recruits were "extremely apprehensive of being infected with the smallpox ... as it proves fatal to many of them."[28]

But through 1776 Washington was hard pressed militarily by the British invasion of New York, and despite his worries about natural smallpox, his prohibition of inoculation remained in place. Congress took the same position issuing a proclamation in 1776 banning inoculation in the Continental Army because of the risks of inoculation.[29]

In addition to the British Army inoculating its fighters against smallpox, their ranks were larger and often filled with survivors of smallpox outbreaks in London or other large population centers and thus immune. In contrast, the Continental Army had significantly fewer fighting men to begin with, many who had grown up in rural areas and had not been exposed to smallpox. As advisable as it might seem to inoculate them all, Washington simply could not spare troops during the fighting season for a possible weeks-long recovery period, even less to countenance a possible three percent mortality rate from the inoculation. The brutal calculus for the Continentals was to hope that enough men would remain healthy or enlist to outweigh those who might be lost to a likely smallpox scourge.

In summer 1776, the British were ready to put down the rebellion. Their target was New York City where there was a large Loyalist population and where the network of waterways allowed the British with its powerful navy the advantage. In the battles around New York in late summer and fall 1776, Washington's inexperience as a commander revealed itself in a series of humiliating American defeats. Yet, to his credit, Washington learned from his mistakes and, at least in part due to good fortune, always kept the army intact.

Accompanied by thousands of German mercenaries, the British force of over 30,000 sailors and soldiers in contrast to 20,000 Continental solders, stormed into New York from the sea, aboard huge fleets from Nova Scotia and the British Isles. To prepare for the massive invasion, Washington had fatefully divided his troops, keeping about half on Manhattan and placing the rest across the East River, in defensive positions in Brooklyn on Long Island. In late August, the British attacked the Brooklyn position first. The king's forces used a nighttime flanking maneuver, caught the Americans totally by surprise, and won a resounding victory. Two weeks later, on September 15th, there was more bad news for Washington. The British invaded Manhattan, overwhelmed a thin American defensive line at the point of attack, and caused the Americans to retreat in panic to upper Manhattan.

For the next few weeks, the remaining 10,000 American troops fortified positions at Harlem Heights in northern Manhattan while the British occupied the rest of the island. In October, rather than attacking the American defenses in upper Manhattan frontally, the British carried out another flanking attack, this time by a water-borne route, forcing the Americans to evacuate Manhattan. Washington's forces retreated twenty-five miles north of New York City to White Plains in Westchester County, where they constructed a strong, hilltop defensive position. Again attacking the American flank, the British dislodged the Americans and forced them to retreat once more, this time across the river to New Jersey, staying barely ahead of the pursuing redcoats. Washington's army just made it to the safety of Pennsylvania, across the Delaware River. In the space of five months, the Continental Army had been defeated time and again. It dwindled from 20,000 in the summer to just 2500 by late December due to enlistments running out, wounds, disease and desertion. Facing a potentially cause-ending crisis, Washington had no time to think about smallpox prevention and inoculation.

In this military crisis, Washington relied upon his resilience, aggressiveness, and bold instincts; he risked it all. On Christmas night 1776, he famously crossed the Delaware River into New Jersey and surprised and defeated isolated, sleepy German regiments in Trenton. It was a desperately needed, one-sided victory for the Americans. Ten days later, Washington was victorious over British regiments in Princeton, New Jersey. These two small, but important victories were noted throughout the Americas and in London and Paris. It was going to be a long war, and the American force with Washington as its commander had a chance.

General Washington's historic decision

In January 1777, the British began wintering in the comfort of New York City while Washington's exhausted men set up an encampment in the village of Morristown, New Jersey. From their strong defensive position there, they were able to counter any British move. They built rude huts for shelter and made the best of wintertime conditions. Washington now had time to ponder the use of inoculation. That month, weighing the pros and cons of inoculation, he did a remarkable about-face. Writing to Director-General of the Medical Department, Dr. William Shippen, he concluded:

> Finding the smallpox to be spreading much, and fearing that no precaution can prevent it from running through the whole of our Army, I have determined that the troops shall be inoculated. The expedient may be attended with some inconvenience and some disadvantages, but yet I trust in its consequences will have the most happy effects ... [S]hould the disorder ... rage with its usual virulence we should have more to dread from it than from the sword of the enemy."[30]

Finally, on February 5, 1777, Washington gave the order for inoculation of his troops in a letter to President of the Continental Congress, John Hancock. The next day, Washington ordered Dr. Shippen to inoculate all recruits in Philadelphia. Five weeks later, Washington designated Philadelphia as an inoculation center as it was not only the American capital and largest American city but also was the major transit center for the army. With these decisions in winter 1777, Washington arranged for his soldiers and new recruits to undergo inoculation and be fully immune in time for the critical campaign of 1777.[31]

By mandating smallpox inoculation for the army, Washington set an early example of "evidence-based public health policy in America."[32] The commander in chief overcame widespread fear and decades of opposition. He showed "both medical foresight and pragmatic leadership" by his courage and willingness to make a difficult decision. Washington was not trained in medicine, but using the analytic tools of a surveyor, he weighed the conflicting data and reached the right decision. It was wintertime with a cessation of fighting. Once Washington had the data and the time, he was able to change his position.

Washington had taken command in July 1775 facing a double crisis from a smallpox outbreak and no coherent prevention strategy. Historians believe that it was the twin American victories in Trenton in last days of December 1776 and in Princeton in first days of January 1777 that saved the cause of independence. While that was correct politically, it was Washington's anguished decision about inoculation that proved "crucial for saving the army, and ultimately the revolution."[33]

---

[1] Freeman. 28-30.

[2] Ibid.

[3] Ibid.

[4] Ibid.

[5] Wehrman, 161-65

[6] Ibid.

[7] Wehrman, 172

[8] Ibid.

Notes, continued

[9] Fees for inoculation were high, reported as high as one to five pounds. At the time, a cow cost about ten pounds. Because of the great demand and large fees, there was medical opportunism. One modification of inoculation was called the Suttonian method after a family that made inoculation a highly profitable business. As noted by one modern historian, "the Suttons were geniuses at self-promotion ... claim[ing] to have an exclusive technique that rendered the effects of the [inoculation] much milder than that of any of their competitors" (Wehrman, 130). They kept their technique secret but likely used an oral mercury compound which was already commonly used by others. In fact, mercury had no benefit and, indeed, commonly led to toxic symptoms. In Marblehead, Massachusetts in the 1770s, investors built an inoculation hospital and charged five pounds, fifteen shillings for the inoculation including the hospital stay during the ensuing illness. The townspeople became angry about the costs, safety and efficacy of the hospital. In January 1774, a group of twenty men "rowed out to the newly built inoculation hospital..., set fire to the despised institution, and burned it to the ground" (Wehrman, 94). There were even outright frauds in the inoculation business. James Latham was a surgeon in the British Army in the 1750s in Quebec. After his service, he entered inoculation practice and made an unsubstantiated claim that he had been trained in inoculation technique by the Suttons. Latham moved to New York in 1770 and made more outlandish claims in his advertisements. Other doctors attacked Latham's statements. One doctor "hoped sensible people would see through Latham's pretenses." Latham was finally exposed as a fraud in 1774 (Wehrman, 134, 159).

[10] Thursfield

[11] Wehrman, 6

[12] What replaced the troublesome inoculation approach was a hallmark innovation by an English country physician, Dr. Edward Jenner, in 1796. Jenner observed that cowpox (a mild infection) on milkmaid Sarah Nelmes's hand made her immune to smallpox. Jenner carried out an experiment in which he deliberately infected an eight-year-old lad, named James Phipps, the son of his gardener. Following the technique of inoculation, Jenner placed material from a cow pox eruption into a scratch in Phipps's arm. When Phipps was subsequently exposed to smallpox, he was protected! Jenner's vaccination technique was ground-breaking. Jenner's process was more effective and much safer than smallpox inoculation. Jenner comes down in medical history as the "Father of Vaccination." Thanks to modern smallpox vaccines, this ancient scourge no longer occurs naturally. The last case of naturally infected smallpox was in a Somali hospital cook in 1977. In laboratories, smallpox virus is kept for research purposes. Today, two vaccines are available if a smallpox outbreak were to occur.

[13] Wehrman, 166

Notes, continued

---

[14] Ibid.

[15] Atkinson, Vol 1, 223

[16] War Office, *17 Monthly Returns*, 17:115 W.O. 17, Vol 1155

[17] Wehrman, 172

[18] Reiss, 88

[19] Blake,127

[20] Wehrman, 173; Jones, Podolsky NEJM, 2281-84

[21] Wehrman, 173; Jones, Podolsky NEJM, 2281-84

[22] Wehrman, 173; Jones, Podolsky NEJM, 2281-84

[23] Wehrman, 173; Jones, Podolsky NEJM, 2281-84

[24] Wehrman, 176-77

[25] Hasselgren World J Surg

[26] Wehrman, 176-77

[27] Washington's War Against Smallpox, website.

[28] Ibid.

[29] Hasselgren World J Surg

[30] Wehrman, 200

[31] Washington's War Against Smallpox, website.

[32] Ibid.

[33] Hasselgren World J Surg

CHAPTER THREE

DR. JAMES TILTON CONTRACTS HOSPITAL FEVER, 1777

Another fighter for the American cause, Dr. James Tilton, like George Washington, literally stood out in a crowd. He was six feet six inches tall at a time when the average American man stood five feet, eight inches and the average British man only five feet, five. Well-educated, honest, generous and even eccentric at times, he would likely have been the center of attention at a social or medical gathering. Serving in the Revolutionary War from its beginning until its end, Dr. Tilton acquired a long and unique perspective. Not only was he a lieutenant in the infantry, a regimental surgeon, and a general hospital physician, but in 1777 Dr. Tilton nearly died from an infection he caught in his military hospital.[1,2] As a direct result, Tilton became an outspoken critic of how the hospitals were run and an advocate for care and hygiene in hospitals.

The campaign for Philadelphia, 1777

To recap, in 1776, the British had won battle after battle but had failed to destroy the American army, and as that fighting season ended the Americans showed surprising resourcefulness in their victories at Trenton and Princeton. Neither of those American victories mattered much militarily, but politically they gave hope for the American cause. They also left British Commander in Chief General Howe seething for revenge.

For the 1777 fighting season, the British embarked on a two-pronged strategy. By traditional European thinking, that strategy should have ended the rebellion. Howe's main army set out from New York on a sea-borne route to capture the American capital, Philadelphia. At the same time, a second British invading force struck from Canada, down the Lake Champlain-Lake George-Hudson River route to separate the New England colonies from the Middle Colonies.[3]. This strategy looked good in theory, but complicated by the distances and conditions of North America, it was flawed—and fatally so. With the two British armies not able to support each other, the royal strategy ended in disaster for them and marked an important turning point of the entire American Revolution as the French subsequently entered the war as American allies.

While part of the British force invaded Philadelphia, the other part was fighting in the fall of 1777 in upstate New York, where their invading army became trapped by a huge American force, numbering about 20,000 at its maximum. After two large battles near Saratoga, New York, the British army of over 6300 men surrendered in entirety in October 1777. American casualties numbered about 330 but were light compared with the British and German total of over 1000 killed and wounded. The French, age-old enemies of the English, had lost Canada in the French and Indian War in the 1760s and were eager to settle the score. Once the French saw a possibility of American military success, they openly jumped in with men, arms, ships, medicines, other supplies, and money. The French Alliance was to prove vital to the success of the American Revolution.

In the Philadelphia campaign, the main British army wound up dealing two severe blows to Washington's main American force, now enhanced by enlistments and supplemented by regiments from other stations (such as along the Hudson). Sailing from New York, General Howe's large army landed at the head of Chesapeake Bay in late August and began the march to Philadelphia, sixty miles away. To defend the American capital Washington chose a defensive position along the Brandywine River at Chadds Ford, in Pennsylvania, about thirty miles southwest of the capital. The British routed the Americans on September 11th. It was the largest single day battle of the war with about 12,000 under Washington versus

18,000 soldiers under Howe. Once again avoiding a frontal attack against established American defenses, the British used a flanking march (similarly to the attack on Long Island the previous August). Washington's army barely escaped only because of a heroic rearguard defense, but it sustained heavy losses. About 250 men were killed and another 600 were wounded. The Continental Army set up hospitals at a safe distance, such as in Princeton, New Jersey, to provide care. Dr. James Tilton was placed in command of the Princeton General Hospital.

Two weeks later, the British marched into Philadelphia without firing a shot. Yet, Washington was not done and attacked the British position in Germantown, outside the American capital, in early October. Although the attack began well for the Americans, Washington's plan was too complicated, and heavy fog caused delays and confusion. The British had time to regroup and then sent the Americans reeling. American losses were again large: nearly 200 killed, more than 500 wounded, and over 400 captured.

The British army spent the winter in Philadelphia. Washington's army endured the brutal winter of 1777-1778 at what became, in the memory of the war, the hallowed encampment at Valley Forge, nineteen miles outside the capital.

For General Howe, his capture of Philadelphia went for naught. Washington's army remained intact, and after just eight months the British evacuated Philadelphia in spring 1778 to consolidate in New York.

Dr. Tilton's hospital

Dr. James Tilton was exceptionally well prepared to command the new general hospital established in Princeton to care for the hundreds of wounded and sick from the 1777 campaign. Born in Delaware in 1745, Tilton served as an apprentice under a prominent physician in Dover.

Apprenticeships in the colonies were three to seven years long. Some apprentices paid a fee which could reach as high as “approximately $100 annually.”[4] There was no standard curriculum and “little book learning”.[5] The apprentice learned under the eye of his mentor with duties that included preparing medicines, spreading plasters, dressing wounds, and attending calls in the night with his master. The apprentice, sometimes starting as young as fifteen years old, might also serve as the master’s “house boy,” messenger, and stable boy. The master provided teaching, moral guidance, and use of his medical books. The apprentice often studied under a relative, suggesting that the relationship was commonly caring and supportive.

In keeping with the loose structure of the system, there were no standard criteria for acceptance into an apprenticeship, giving rise to a quip attributed to Dr. Benjamin Rush that the only prerequisite was “the ability to stand the sight of blood.”[6] In addition, there was no accreditation process for the apprenticeships. The Colony of Massachusetts attempted “regulation by issuing a certificate of proficiency for completion of an approved apprenticeship.” There were no licensing examinations. When Massachusetts tried to establish licensing in the Eighteenth Century, it was thwarted as it was seen as “an effort to place a monopoly on medicine”.[7]

Tilton, having completed his apprenticeship but desiring more formal education, enrolled in the first class at the new medical school in Philadelphia. Called the College of Philadelphia, it was the first medical school in the American colonies, founded in 1765. (It later became the University of Pennsylvania School of Medicine.) Tilton initially received the degree of Bachelor of Medicine in 1768 and then his Medical Doctor in 1771. He was successful in his medical practice in Dover when the war broke out in April 1775.

The twenty-nine-year-old Tilton responded by becoming an infantry lieutenant in the Delaware militia. As the war heated up, a Delaware Regiment of the Continental Army was organized, under Colonel John Haslet, also a physician. On January 16, 1776, James Tilton became the regimental surgeon accompanying this heroic unit in battles throughout the New York campaign at Brooklyn, White Plains, Trenton and Princeton. The Delaware Regiment was "practically wiped out" after the heavy 1776 fighting season. For the rest of winter 1777, Tilton cared for the sick and wounded of his regiment in a hospital set up in Wilmington, Delaware.

In April 1777, with Tilton's excellent medical and surgical reputation spreading within the army, Congress put him in charge of smallpox inoculations for Continental soldiers reporting to a center in Virginia. He remained in this position until September when he was called to command the new general hospital in Princeton.

At the Princeton hospital, Tilton noted, "(with) the sick and wounded, flowing promiscuously without restraint into the hospital, it soon became infectious and was attended by great mortality." He must not have been surprised. He would later write, "Not only hospitals filled with sick, but whole encampments of well men may become infectious. War and pestilence are proverbially connected together."[8] The cause of most of the deaths was a disease then variously called jail, hospital, ship, or camp fever, known subsequently as typhus.[9]

From his medical studies and his own observations, Tilton would have known how to diagnose typhus. He knew of the works of Sir John Pringle,[10] the brilliant Eighteenth-Century British physician who is recognized as the "Father of Military Medicine," and likely would have read Pringle's description of typhus, written in 1750:

> Some preserve their senses, allowing for confusion and stupor through the whole course of the disease till recovery; few keep them till death... The confusion of the head often rises to

> delirium, especially at night, but rarely turns to rage... There are certain spots which are frequent but not inseparable attendants of the fever... They are of the petechial kind, of an obscure red colour, paler than the measles, not raised above the skin, of no regular shape, but confluent.... These petchiae ... appear as early as the fourth or fifth day, and at other times as late as the fourteenth".[11]

Although no one at the time knew exactly how typhus spread, it was clear that hospitals were terribly contagious places even for the medical staff. Tilton wrote, poignantly, "More surgeons died, in the American service, in proportion to their numbers, than officers of the line, strong evidence that infection is more dangerous in military life than the weapons of war."[12]

Then from exposure in his own hospital teeming with disease, Tilton tells us, "I caught the jail fever myself and narrowly escaped with my life." Although he does not give his specific symptoms, his course most likely would have begun after incubation of eight to sixteen days, with an abrupt chill followed by high fever, headache, and leg and back pains. Since he was so ill, he probably had delirium for part of the time. His distinguishing rash would have consisted of rose-colored spots which evolved into petechiae (small spots with bleeding in the skin). Infestations with vermin were common in the unhygienic hospital conditions, and upon close inspection Dr. Tilton's body would almost certainly have harbored what we recognize today as disease-carrying lice. Other doctors no doubt treated Tilton with the recommended treatments of the day: bleedings, emetics, cathartics, and for pain, opium preparations. We may presume that Tilton was sick for two to three weeks when his illness probably ended in a dramatic resolving event referred to as a "crisis" in which he would have awakened after a deep sleep feeling better and clear minded.

His course must have been debilitating. He wrote, "After a tedious illness, I got leave to return home for the recovery of my health".[13] Lucky indeed was Dr. Tilton for the mortality rate from typhus back then as high as fifty percent.

Crowding, Contagion. And Death

En route to his home in Delaware, Tilton inspected other general hospitals. Based upon his excellent medical education for the time, his own extensive experience, and quite possibly the writings about crowding and hospitals of other doctors, Tilton had become an expert in hospital infections, especially typhus.

One book perhaps available to him was written the year before by his contemporary, Dr. John Jones of New York.[14] In Jones' descriptions, Tilton might have read that the great cities of Europe with large populations and polluted air were terribly unhealthy and that the huge city hospitals were even worse. From his personal observations in Europe, Jones vividly called populous cities "the graves of the human species," and "the large and crowded hospitals, generally built in them, may with equal truth and propriety be deemed the lazarettos or pest-houses of most of the unfortunate persons who ... are carried into these charities." Based on his visits as a young physician to the great hospitals in London and Paris, Jones wrote that the long wards were scenes of dense crowding, horror and misery. Beds were placed in triple rows with four to six patients per bed. More than once, Jones wrote, that on morning rounds, he found the dead lying with the living. There were so many patients, so packed together, that it was "almost impossible ... to bestow timely assistance upon every individual"[15].

Some clinical textbooks were certainly available in the medical school libraries, and perhaps as a student, if not later, Tilton may have had access to a copy of Sir John Pringle's 1750 hallmark book, *Observations on the Nature and Cure of Hospital and Jayl Fevers*. Pringle described Eighteenth-Century British military hospitals as suffering the same plight as the big European city hospitals owing to great masses of men and unsanitary conditions. He vividly described military hospitals as "filled with the poisonous effluvia of sores, mortifications, dysenteric and other putrid excrements," and he correctly attributed many hospital deaths to "filth, crowding, and utter lack of hygiene".[16] From his first-hand experience in European wars, Pringle gave a horrifying picture of his large hospital where there were the wounded as well as 1500 sick. "The air became so much vitiated, that not only the rest of the patients, but the apothecaries, nurses, and others employed in the hospital ... were infected." Initially most of sick had dysentery, but "to this was added a still more alarming distemper, namely the Jail or Hospital fever," which he attributed to "the common effects of foul air from crowds and animal corruption".[17]

Thus, as fully prepared to do hospital inspections as anyone in the Continental Army, Dr. Tilton set out from Princeton. Because the British occupied Philadelphia, Tilton had to take a circuitous route to home in Delaware and visited a hospital set up in the house of a religious order in Bethlehem, Pennsylvania (seventy miles from Philadelphia). There, as a result of the Battles at Brandywine and Germantown, he found 700 American sick and wounded packed into the hospital which was considered crowded with just 450 men. Typhus rampaged through the wards, killing 300 men in three months. Even the medical staff was cursed. Ten of eleven surgeons and mates caught typhus, and one died. The hospital's three stewards all became ill, and two died. The orderlies and nurses all became afflicted with typhus as well. The disease even spread to the brothers of the religious order, seven of whom developed fatal cases. By the time the Bethlehem general hospital closed in June 1778,1500 soldiers had been admitted, many initially for dysentery or respiratory infections. Debilitated from these conditions, the men were ripe for typhus, which spread from man to man. Of those admitted, fully one in three died. Two hundred North Carolinians died there, representing half of all the state's casualties in the war. When Dr. Benjamin Rush later investigated the mortality rate at the Bethlehem hospital, he attributed the high rate to dense crowding and contaminated air.[18] Indeed, the Bethlehem Hospital was especially stricken by disease, but even in less crowded general hospitals the death rate was appreciable. In a best case, early in the war, there was the Cambridge hospital in1775 with a mortality of just six per-cent. However, in New York City in 1776 when the army reached over 20,000 men, hospital mortality rose to ten percent, and in the winter of 1777-1778 in Pennsylvania and New Jersey, when influenza and pneumonia added to the dangers, the hospital mortality climbed to twenty-five percent.[19]

In the Continental Army, the general hospitals were intended to be jewels in the crown of the Medical Department, but they fared no better than British general hospitals or large city hospitals of the day. From dangerous overcrowding, improper hygiene, and poor ventilation, disease especially typhus ran rampant. Dr. Benjamin Rush, who in 1777 wrote a pamphlet on preserving the health of soldiers, lamented that the general hospitals "robbed the country of more citizens than the sword".[20]

Like Doctor Rush, whose manual on the subject will be addressed in Chapter Four, Tilton was a champion of cleanliness. Stating what today seems obvious, he recommended that the "same bedding should never be used for more than one patient without cleansing" but his suggestion for the best method of cleansing was to turn the bunks "out of doors to receive the full benefit of air, rain, frost, & c." It was even necessary for him to add that "all manner of clothing should be washed" and that "the utmost care should be taken to remove all excrementitious matter from the wards, so as to leave no smell behind them".[21] Tilton reinforced the need for "separating those ill of fevers, fluxes, &c. from the wounded and such as have only slight topical affectations." He attested that "many a fine fellow have I seen brought into the hospital, for slight syphilitic affections and carried out dead of a hospital fever".[22]

In blunt language, Tilton decried the crowding and contagion in the general hospitals and claimed that they "swallowed up at least one half of our army, owing to a fatal tendency in the system to throw all the sick of the army into the general hospital".[23] From their horrific descriptions, medical champions of better care—heroes like Pringle in England and Rush and Tilton in America—laid the foundation for infection control and military hygiene, as explored in Chapter Four.

---

[1] AMEDD, Surgeons General, "Tilton", website

[2] Tilton, 29

[3] The thirteen colonies were grouped as New England (New Hampshire, Massachusetts, Rhode Island, and Connecticut), Middle colonies (New York, Pennsylvania, New Jersey, and Delaware), and the Southern colonies (Maryland, Virginia, North Carolina, South Carolina, and Georgia). Vermont was not an original colony.

[4] Griesemer

[5] Rosenberg

[6] Ibid.

[7] Turley

[8] Tilton, 32

[9] Typhus has been a scourge throughout history and remained a cause of great epidemics in large European cities well into the Nineteenth Century. In the early Twentieth Century, the history of typhus was described as "written in those dark pages of the world's story which tell of the grievous visitations of mankind by ... misery of every kind" (Osler, 51). In modern times, typhus is rarely seen, with outbreaks occurring where populations are clustered together amidst poor hygiene as in war, famine, and refugee camps. It is a disease caused by the micro-organism *Rickettsia prowazekii* and is spread by the human body louse. Laboratory confirmation of the diagnosis is available through blood tests to detect specific antibodies. When treated early with the common antibiotic doxycycline, the course is shortened, complications prevented, and death avoided.

[10] Born in 1707 to a family of baronets and academics, John Pringle was educated at the University of Edinburgh and received his Doctor of Medicine from Leyden, Netherlands in 1730. He returned to Edinburgh to practice medicine and teach moral philosophy at the university. In 1742, Pringle

Notes, continued

served as a surgeon to the British forces in Europe where he was saw the inhumane treatment of prisoners of war and the wounded of both sides. Pringle advocated for cleanliness, adequate ventilation, and good hygiene—all pillars of infection control today. He had a distinguished career, serving as President of the Royal Society for six years and as Physician Extraordinary to the King. Pringle died in London in 1782 at age 75 years.

[11] Editorial, "Sir John Pringle (1707-1782)—Military Physician and Hygienist," *JAMA* 190, no. 9 (November 1964): 113

[12] Tilton, 64

[13] Ibid, 20

[14] John Jones, Plain Concise Practical Remarks, on the Treatment of Wounds and Fractures (Philadelphia: Robert Bell, 1776).

[15] Jones, Plain Concise Practical Remarks,102-104

[16] Editorial, "Sir John Pringle," 114.

[17] Tilton, 31

[18] Reiss, 187-88

[19] Ibid.

[20] Reiss, 40

[21] Tilton, 21

[22] Ibid, 54-55

[23] Ibid, 13

CHAPTER FOUR

DR. BENJAMIN RUSH PRESERVES THE HEALTH OF THE ARMY, 1777

Like Tilton, but even more influential, Doctor Benjamin Rush (1745-1813) was certainly the most remarkable American physician of the revolution. He was handsome and "spellbindingly sure of himself ... possessing an "outsized ego." Rush's "capacious mind was paired with a fast, glib tongue".[1] Tireless, he slept just four to five hours a night. To feed his intellect and energy, he acquired vast educational and personal experiences in America, Britain and France. In his expansive career, he served not only in high medical posts but also was a leader in Congress and one of the disproportionate number of physicians who were signers of the Declaration of Independence.

Rush was born near Philadelphia as one of seven children into a prominent Pennsylvania family, which had left England with William Penn in 1683.[2] His father, a farmer, landowner, and gunsmith, died in 1751 leaving his mother to support the family. Rush was able to attend The College of New Jersey (later Princeton University) and became an apprentice for five years under the highly respected physician, Dr. John Redman, who received his medical education at the University of Leyden in the Netherlands and then worked at Guy's Hospital in London before returning to Philadelphia. Redman was a man of good sense and achieved distinction including first President of the College of Physicians of Philadelphia and member of the prestigious American Philosophical Society. No doubt Rush acquired many of his attitudes from his mentorship under Redman.

In the summer of 1766, Rush sought more formal medical education, sailed to Europe, and soon obtained his medical degree at the University of Edinburgh. Afterwards, he had a head-spinning time for a young man. Most importantly, in 1768, he came under the mentorship of Benjamin Franklin, then an American representative in England. Through Franklin, Rush met the Continent's great figures of medicine, letters, and the arts. He befriended Doctor John Fothergill, an English Quaker known for his writings on plant biology, epidemic sore throat, and angina, and fellow Pennsylvanian, painter Benjamin West. He was introduced to the famed portraitist, Sir Joshua Reynolds, and attended a dinner with Oliver Goldsmith, James Boswell, and Samuel Johnson. He met the noted political thinker and orator John Wilkes.[3] Rush gained additional medical experience by traveling to Paris, a trip financed by Franklin. Returning to America, Rush opened his practice in Philadelphia, enhancing his reputation by providing care without pay to the city's poor.[4] In 1769, at just twenty-four years of age but aided by Franklin's endorsement, he was appointed to the faculty as Professor of Chemistry at the new medical school, The College of Philadelphia, just four years after it opened.[5]

Rush's interest in politics began in 1774 when he met John Adams, who was in Philadelphia for the First Continental Congress. In September 1775, Rush became physician and surgeon to Pennsylvania's small fleet plying the Delaware River and by early 1776 was a member of the city's radical movement. Although not yet a member of Congress when the vote for independence was taken on July 2, 1776, Rush was appointed to Congress a few weeks later and then became a signer of the Declaration of Independence.

Earlier in January 1776, Rush had married Julia Stockton, the sixteen-year-old daughter of Richard Stockton, another signer of the Declaration. Together, Benjamin and Julia Rush had thirteen children, but a family tragedy struck, all too common for the times, as four died in the first year of life. It was a time of high infant mortality (up to thirty percent by age five years), mainly from infections.

During the war, Rush served in the administrative post of Surgeon General of the Continental Army's Middle Department for several months in 1777. Because of his stellar reputation for medical skills, he was called upon in January 1777 to care for the mortally wounded General Hugh Mercer in Princeton and in September 1777 for the wounded and dying men lying on the Brandywine battlefield.

A product of the Enlightenment, Rush was farsighted. Later in life, he worked with Franklin to abolish slavery, and he supported the education of women. One of his lasting medical contributions was in advocating humane care for the mentally ill, earning him the title of "The Father of American Psychiatry."

Mentored by Franklin, articulate and brilliant, but also pragmatic, Benjamin Rush was just the American physician to take on the prevailing lax attitudes towards to health of soldiers.

Personal hygiene in Eighteenth Century North America

To understand Rush's challenge and to appreciate his contributions to medicine by insisting on hygienic practices, it helps to get a picture of what personal hygiene was like 250 years ago for townsfolk and farm families in North America. For the Eighteenth-Century soldier, living in the field during the fighting season in and in crowded encampments during the winter, hygiene seemed a distant afterthought.

In Eighteenth-Century populations, oral hygiene was still crude. Bristle toothbrushes, an age-old invention of the Chinese, had begun to make their appearance in parts of the Western world, but were not yet common in colonial North America. Some people in the colonies scrubbed their teeth with salt. Others used burnt breadcrumbs, pulverized eggshells or oyster shells, baking soda, alum, vinegar, and even tobacco. To freshen the breath, chewing mint or parsley was popular. Many probably practiced no oral hygiene. Before toothbrushes, colonials used frayed twigs or towels for scrubbing their teeth.[6]

With preventive dental care so poor, tooth decay and cavities were universal and were treated by extraction with a pliers or forceps.[7] Poor oral hygiene had implications in military readiness. Soldiers with active mouth and gum infection were likely more susceptible to killer diseases. Further, infantrymen needed two opposing teeth to bite the paper end from the cartridges. Even young men might have lost most of their teeth and thus not be able to serve, at least not in the infantry.

Two hundred-fifty years ago, no one had running water, and soap was precious. After toiling on the farm or in a sweaty shop, most everyone simply sponged the hands and face in basins of water, perhaps heated in the kitchen. Even among upper class civilians in colonial North America, bathing was a major affair, requiring lugging the empty wooden tub from the laundry house, hoisting water from the well, heating the water in the fireplace, and filling the tub.[8]

In towns and cities, commercial soap makers (called "soap boilers") had been established in colonial America since the 1600s, but most soap was homemade even through the early 1800s. In the Eighteenth Century, the homemade or commercial process was messy and time-consuming. Soap was made by boiling wood ash (containing the alkali chemicals potash or pearlash) with rendered animal fat.[9] (The chemical process, called saponification, is still the fundamental principle in soap production today.) Rendering animal fat (that is, cleaning it of the meat) was a smelly job. The mixture of rendered fat and lye was boiled in a kettle for six to eight hours. When allowed to cool, the product was a brownish, gelatinous, slippery substance, called "soft soap." It was stored in barrels and ladled out as needed. For more convenient storage and transport, soft soap could be made into hard soap by adding salt. This soap product was then cut into bars. However, because salt in colonial America was expensive, hard soap was less commonly used.

Most Americans had few changes of clothes, perhaps just a single set. The interaction between sweat and skin bacteria caused what we call today "body odor." Because wool, the main fabric for clothing, needed a long time to dry, outfits were infrequently washed. It all resulted in most people smelling bad. Further, with typhus, for example, spread by lice, unwashed, infested clothing spread disease.

Health and hygiene in the army

Military life made things even worse. It was a health powder keg. There were large masses of unkempt men and camp followers crowded together in filth. When Washington took command around Boston in July 1775, he found the army so dirty that he approved them bathing in the Charles River. The next summer in Manhattan, the army numbering 20,000 was packed on Harlem Heights. Five thousand men were encamped at the forward lines on the southern lip, and thrice that number were deployed farther north up the heights. In the hot and humid weather, the work of building earthen fortifications and manhandling field cannons was exhausting. Their uniforms of either of linen or of wool became soaked in sweat. Frequent body washing and changes of clothing were just not practical for so large an army encamped on the plateau. There was limited washing, mainly of the hands and face and in warm weather perhaps a swim in a nearby creek or river. Finding supplies of soap, in the quantities needed for a large army, plagued the army's commissary even though Congress had established the soap ration as early as 1775. (See Table 4-1.)

Imagine the huge amount of excrement that an army of 20,000 men produced each day. As a matter of sanitation, latrines (also called vaults or necessaries) were dug around the camps, and they were supposed to be covered with fresh earth daily. However, soldiers commonly avoided use of the latrines in favor of a less foul and more convenient spot in the trees, but if caught, there was punishment by public lashing.

Wintertime brought additional disease prevention challenges. Proper shelter, adequate warmth, and fresh food were limited. During the heroic winter at Valley Forge (1777-1778), the army remained in tents for weeks before they were able to build their crude log huts. Even when completed, these shelters were crowded, drafty, and cold, perfect set-ups for typhus, dysentery, and pneumonia. Warm clothing was in short supply. In February 1778, one-third of the men in the Valley Forge encampment were unfit for duty owing to a lack of winter coats and footwear.[10] Feeding an army of 12,000 was a monumental task. For nearly the entire winter of 1778, food supplies ran short. In the winter two years later—1779-1780—at Morristown, New Jersey, food supply was so short that hungry troops resorted to stealing from nearby farms. In response, Washington resorted to ordering floggings for soldiers who were caught plundering.[11]

From the foul odor arising from the hundreds of improperly covered latrines, the encampments could be smelled from far away. The entire army stank and was a set up for epidemic disease. Yet, among the officer corps, there was a complacency, a strangely indifferent attitude about these foreboding, unhealthy conditions. It was time for Dr. Rush to preserve the army.

Dr. Rush gives directions

In 1777, Doctor Benjamin Rush stepped boldly into the precarious health morass. Under order of the Board of War, Rush, who was then Physician General to the Military Hospitals of the United States, published *Directions for Preserving the Health of Soldiers*. Rush began by succinctly pointing to the interwoven strategic, physical, and moral high stakes:

> Fatal experience has taught the people of America that a greater proportion of men have perished with sickness in our armies than have fallen by the sword ... The gallant youth who had torn himself from the arms of his parents, or the partner of his joys ... was often forced from the scene of action

> and glory by the attack of a fever, and obligated to languish for days or weeks in a hospital; and, at last to close his eyes, deprived of ... the thoughts of ending his life in the arms of victory, or in an act of just resentment against the enemies of the liberties of his country... The munificence of the congress has made the most ample provision for lessening the calamities of war from sickness in their armies, and, if possible to prevent it altogether.[12]

He urged the line officers of the army to "enforce the most salutary plan, and precepts for preserving the health of the soldiers".[13] He argued passionately for implementation of preventative measures because "the munificence of the congress, and the skill of physicians and surgeons, will avail but little in preventing mortality without the concurrence of the officers of the army." Rush's pamphlet was so complete that it influenced American military hygiene through the Civil War seventy-five years later.

From the perspective of the Twenty-First Century, Rush's directions seem simple and straight-forward, but for the time they were not. Indeed, from reading Rush's far-sighted exhortations, he believed he had to do a great deal of convincing to shake the line officers from their indifference about health and hygiene. Rush was not the first physician to write about preserving the health of the armies. Twenty-five years before Rush's *Directions*, the science of military medicine was founded through the pioneering work of the eminent Scottish physician, Sir John Pringle, who in 1752 published *Observations on Diseases of the Army.*

In America, Rush took up Pringle's banner of prevention. Rush identified five "particulars" for preserving the health of soldiers. First, noting that *dress* had a great influence on a soldier's health, Rush lamented that uniforms were "chiefly in linen." It was well known, he wrote, that perspiration "attached itself to linen, and afterwards by mixing with rain, is predisposed to form miasmata (unhealthy smells or vapors), which produce fevers." He advocated wearing flannel shirts under the linen to absorb the perspiration. He further hypothesized that long, uncombed hair collected perspiration which "by becoming putrid produces diseases." Rush recommended wearing it "thin and short."

Second, Rush advocated for a *diet* chiefly of vegetables which were to be "well cooked." Rush's dietary advice was a far-thinking proposal since in 1775 Congress had established rather unhealthy rations for a soldier: meat, usually beef including bone, fat and gristle, or salt fish; bread or flour to make firecakes (made from flour, water, meat and gristle); dried peas or beans ; rice or cornbread daily; and spruce beer or cider or two ounces of spirits per day.[14] Fresh vegetables and fruits and fresh meat were not part of the regular ration but were provided when available. See Table 4-1.

Table 4-1. Ration for Each Soldier, by Resolution of Congress, November 1775*

1 lb. of beef [typically salted or preserved], or ¾ lb. pork, or 1 lb. salt fish, per day
1 lb. of bread or flour per day
3 pints of "pease," or beans per week, or vegetables equivalent, at one dollar per bushel for "pease" or beans
1 pint of milk per man per day, or at the rate of 1/72 of a dollar
1 half pint of Rice, or 1 pint of Indian meal [cornbread] per man per week
1 quart of spruce beer** or cyder per man per day, or nine gallons of Molasses per company of 100 men per week
3 lb. candles to 100 men per week for guards
24 lb. of soft soap or 8 lb. hard soap for 100 men per week

* Source: Washington Papers, washingtonpapers.org/resources/articles/supply-problems-plagued-the-continental-army-from-the-start, Accessed August 8, 2025.[15]

** Spruce beer, made with the buds and needles of spruce trees, was popular either as an alcoholic or non-alcoholic beverage in North America. It turned out that it contained Vitamin C, the preventive and treatment for scurvy.

Rush railed against "the custom of drinking spiritous liquors, which prevails so generally in our army." He noted that "the use of rum ... lays the foundation of fevers, fluxes, jaundices, and most of the diseases which occur in military hospitals." Rather, he argued for the health benefits of "plentiful draughts of milk and water."

Third, Rush advocated for *cleanliness* for in its absence an army as numerous as "blades of grass on the continent of America ..." would be reduced "in two or three campaigns to a handful of men." Accordingly, he wrote that soldiers should be obligated to wash their hands and face daily and the whole body two or three times a week, especially in summer. Rush further directed that "frequent changes of linen [clothing] are indispensably necessary," and unless strictly regarded, "all our pains to preserve the health of our soldiers, will be to no purpose." He even had to state that "great care" should be taken in washing "the vessels in which [the soldier] cooks his victuals" after each meal. Rush warned against "too many soldiers ... crowd[ing] into the same tent or quarter." He correctly identified that "gaol fever" (typhus) was the "offspring" of crowding, but he thought it was spread by "perspiration and respiration of human bodies brought into a compass too narrow to be diluted."

Soldiers often slept with a blanket on a bed of straw or hay. Rush recommended changing the straw often and exposing the blanket to the sun daily to "prevent the perspiration from becoming morbid and dangerous by accumulating upon it." The commanding officer, Rush stated, "should take the utmost care never to suffer a soldier to sleep, or even to sit down in a wet blanket or upon wet straw." As his last recommendation for cleanliness, Rush warned that "the environs of each tent, and of the camp in general ... should be kept perfectly clean of the offals of animals and of filth of all kinds."

Fourth, Rush addressed the formation of the *encampment*. There was no purpose, he advised line officers, in disposing the troops "where marshes and mill-ponds let loose intermittent fevers [malaria] upon them." Rush correctly observed the ill effects of encampments near marshes. At the time, he blamed the marshy air *per se*. It was not until one hundred years later that science identified the true cause as the disease-carrying mosquitoes living in proximity to the water. Further, to guard against "the effects of those offal matters," he urged "frequently changing the spot of an encampment." Rush then warned against "unnecessary" fatigue, by carrying out daily exercises in the cool of the morning and evening in summer and by relieving sentries "often" in very hot, cold and rainy weather. To restore and preserve the purity of air, he advised the "singular efficacy" of "fire and smoke of wood, as also the burning of sulfur, and the explosion of gunpowder," despite how irritating these fumes must have been to the lungs.

Finally, as "idleness is the bane of a soldier," he recommended regular exercise. "Nothing can be more destructive to the lives of men," he wrote, than passing "from the extremes of labour to the extremes of idleness."

The good doctor concluded his directions with "a few hints which are worthy of the attention of the gentlemen of the army". These paragraphs were a passionate appeal to the officers to adhere to his directions. Rush began with reason and cajoling. Because the principal duty of an officer, in time of war, "should be to save the blood of his men," it was equally important to save their lives in the encampment as well as on the battlefield. His appeal turned to heavy emotional motivation.

> Nature has given the Americans strength; and the cause of liberty has given them principle above the common soldier of any army on the face of the earth. The blame, therefore, will only be yours, if they are not made superior to them in all the arts which improve and adorn a soldier's person and character.
>
> Lastly, consider that your country and posterity look up to you for the preservation of the only means of establishing the liberties of America.... All our hopes, therefore, are in our army.... Consider further, that there is scarcely a soldier under your command who has not a mother, a wife, a sister, or a child.... Whenever your duty requires that you should attend to the health of your men, imagine you see *one* or perhaps *all* of their female ... connexions standing at the door of your tents or quarters, and beseeching you ... to attend to everything ... necessary for the preservation of their health and lives.[16]

Doctor Rush made it seem no more than a matter of will for the officers to comply with his directions to preserve the army's health. But conditions of crowding, exhaustion, exposure to extremes of weather, and poor nutrition were well beyond the control of individual officers. Finally, underlying all the supply problems was the weakness of Congress. Despite Rush's praise for the "munificence" of Congress, the representatives had endless difficulties in raising money for the war effort, in getting financial credit, and in obtaining wholesome food and medical supplies.

The principles of military hygiene and disease prevention were established in the late Eighteenth Century, long before the scientific basis was known. The great writings of Doctors Pringle and Rush showed how to apply the principles, but implementation was thwarted by organizational, logistical, financial, and psychological obstacles, and by Mother Nature herself. Failed implementation set the stage for rampant disease.

Rush's pamphlet was a Herculean step forward, but despite the wisdom of Rush's five directives, it was simply impractical for medical and line officers to apply them completely to an army in the field or in a wintertime garrison. Nonetheless, did Rush's pamphlet, published in 1777, have an impact? At least one observation indicates that it did. Between the winter of 1778-1779 at Valley Forge and the winter of 1779-1780 at Morristown, New Jersey— one of the harshest in Eighteenth Century North America, camp hygiene improved greatly, and fewer than one hundred men died of disease or exposure, a mortality rate twenty-fold less than at Valley Forge. Although there may have been other causes also contributing to the better health outcomes, Rush deserves credit. In a crisis, vision and leadership are essential.

---

[1] Stephen Fried, Rush: Revolution, Madness, and the Visionary Doctor Who Became a Founding Father (New York: Crown, 2018), 9.

[2] Fried, *Rush*, 15-16.

[3] John Wilkes Booth, the infamous American actor and assassin of Abraham Lincoln, was named after Eighteenth Century John Wilkes as the Booth family considered the famous English statesman a remote relative.

[4] Gifford, 25.

[5] Fried, *Rush*, 73.

[6] Commercial toothpaste was not introduced until the 1820s.

[7] The George Washington Foundation, "Dental Care in Early America," *Lives & Legacies* (blog), September 2, 2015, accessed August 8, 2025, livesandlegaciesblog.org/2015/09/ 02/dental-care-in-early-america. Also, Loomis Road Dental Center, "Colonial Dental Treatments," loomisroaddental.com/colonial-dental-treatments, accessed August 8, 2025.

[8] Edwards Park, "To Bathe or Not to Bathe: Coming Clean in Colonial America," *Colonial Williamsburg Journal*, Autumn 2000, accessed December 18, 2025, research.colonialwilliamsburg.org/foundation/ journal/Autumn00/bathe.cfm.

Notes, continued

[9] Colonial Soap Making, website.

[10] Rick Atkinson, The Fate of the Day: The War for America, Fort Ticonderoga to Charleston, 1777–1780, vol. 2 of The Revolution Trilogy (New York: Crown, 2025), 293-97.

[11] Atkinson, *The Fate of the Day*, 559-62.

[12] Rush, 3.

[13] Rush,13.

[14] US Army Revolutionary War 250th Commemoration, website.

[15] Washington Papers, website.

[16] Rush, 13-14.

CHAPTER FIVE

DR. JOHN JONES ADVANCES MILITARY SURGERY, 1776

For Dr. John Jones, Professor of Surgery in New York, the decision about separating from England was not easy. Like most colonists, he undoubtedly felt a loyalty to the Crown. His Welsh ancestors had come to Pennsylvania nearly a hundred years before the revolution, and he enjoyed the security of living in British North America. Indeed, he had already served the Mother Country during the French and Indian War when he was a young surgeon in the New York militia. Yet a decade of Parliament's economic and political oppression pushed him to side with those favoring independence. Still, Jones was not a radical and condemned the extremists for their boycotts. On June 20, 1775, two months after Lexington and Concord and three days after Bunker Hill, he learned of Washington's appointment as commander in chief. He welcomed the news but did not rule out reconciliation. He wrote to a colleague, "If they [a Royal Commission] come quickly, to offer you something like a chart blanche, perhaps we may have peace upon the footing of reconciliation, otherwise, from the rising spirit and temper of the people, I presume you will have under necessity of declaring ourselves the High and Mighty States of the Thirteen United Colonies."[1]

A year later, after the signing of the Declaration of Independence and the British capture of Manhattan, Surgeon John Jones "was forced to actively take a side [of the patriots] in the growing conflict."[2] A life-long bachelor, he had no family responsibilities and headed off to war. For men of all ranks and stations with families to provide for, the decision to respond to the call for service was difficult.

Dr. Jones learns about medicine

Almost from birth, it seemed, Jones was preparing for this historic rendezvous. Born on Long Island in 1729, both his father and grandfather were physicians. He had his early education in a private school in New York. At age eighteen years, he decided to follow in his family's medical footsteps. With no medical schools in the colonies then, he took an apprenticeship in Philadelphia for three years with Dr. Thomas Cadwalader, a cousin who turned out to be an excellent medical mentor. Cadwalader had himself been an apprentice under Jones's father, subsequently traveled to Europe, and received his medical doctorate at the University of Rheims in France. Of his own apprenticeship, Jones wrote, "Both in physic and morals [I received] the best and earliest lessons of my life."[3]

To pursue more formal medical education, Jones followed Dr. Cadwalader's path and earned his medical doctorate in 1751 at Rheims, France. For his required thesis, he prepared a paper entitled, *Observations on Wounds*, which would serve as the basis for his 1776 book (*Plain Concise Practical Remarks on the Treatment of Wounds and Fractures*), the first medical text published in North America. After graduation, Jones gleaned first-hand experience by meeting a leading French surgeon (Claude Le Cat, who perfected operations to remove bladder stones) and visiting Paris's immense hospital, the charity hospital Hotel-Dieu (House of God). Jones's observations there stayed with him his entire career and influenced his future views on hospital care and design.

With these skills, Jones returned to New York, opened his surgical practice, and quickly became known as a lithotomist (a surgeon who removed painful and obstructing bladder stones). So skilled and facile, Jones could perform the stone removal in just over a minute. The surgery, performed without anesthesia, involved making an incision between the anus and scrotum to reach and remove the bladder stone.

When the French and Indian War broke out, Jones rallied to the colors and volunteered with the New York militia. During a battle in 1755 in upper New York State, the French commander was wounded four times. So wide was Jones's reputation already that the enemy French commander, Baron d'Escoux, requested that Jones treat him. Jones saved d'Escoux's life, further enhancing his status as one of the most prominent American surgeons.[4] At the time, it was not uncommon for surgeons of one force to treat the wounded of the enemy if they were not overwhelmed by their own casualties. Indeed, as a humanitarian measure, during a mid-Eighteenth-Century European war, a novel convention signed by commanders of the English, French and Austrian forces established the neutrality of hospitals. The noted English physician John Pringle wrote that hospitals should be considered as "sanctuaries for the sick, and mutually protected."[5]

Jones seemed to do it all. After the French and Indian War, he returned to New York City where he and four other distinguished physicians established a medical school at King's College (later Columbia University College of Physicians and Surgeons) in 1767. It was only the second medical school in the colonies. The first was the College of Philadelphia, which opened in 1765. Jones also worked industriously for a royal charter to form New York Hospital. The charter was granted in 1771, and Jones was appointed to the staff in 1774. Based on his harrowing observations at Hotel Dieu, Jones was able to influence the design of the new hospital limiting the number of beds to eight in each ward and allowing for adequate ventilation.1 This hospital burned to the ground during the great Fire of September 1775 and was not rebuilt until 1791.

The first American medical text

And yet there was more—much more—to John Jones's extraordinary contributions to surgery and the war. In 1776, Jones published his short (114 pages) book, *Plain Concise*

Practical Remarks ..., that would have lasting effect on surgical care during the Revolutionary War and beyond. Jones dedicated his hallmark book to his mentor, Dr. Thomas Cadwalader. Reflecting his own patriotic views, Jones's dedication read in part:

> The present calamitous situation of this once happy country ... demands the aid and assistance of every virtuous citizen; ... every man has it in his power to contribute something towards so desirable an end; and if he cannot cure the fatal diseases of his unfortunate country, it will, at least, afford him some consolation, to have poured a little balm into her bleeding wounds...[6]

The book was not a full textbook but a pragmatic manual on treatment of wounds and fractures and was "designed for the Use of young Military and naval Surgeons in North America".[7] He offered guidance to these young surgeons likely to see mass battle casualties for the first time. Jones advised "a liberal education ... graced by the constant practice of attention, tenderness, and humanity." He continued, "A judicious surgeon will always find his powers and abilities of assisting the wretched proportionate to the time he has spent, and the pains he has bestowed in acquiring the proper knowledge of his profession".[8] The qualities Jones identified in a "good Surgeon" reflect the values of the Hippocratic Oath, originally written in ancient Greece. The oath emphasizes the physician's ethical and moral responsibilities, confidentiality, avoiding harm, and doing good. An expression arising from the oath, "first, do no harm," is regularly heard today in medical teaching and care. Finally, Jones advised the corps of young surgeons "to have firm steady hands, and be able to use both alike; a strong clear sight, and above all, a mind calm and intrepid, yet humane and compassionate, avoiding every appearance of terror and cruelty to his patients, amidst the most severe operations."[9]

When John Jones wrote his book, surgery was a gruesome business. Surgical operations were necessarily few and brief. Military surgery was limited to treatment of gunshot wounds and stabbings, setting of fractures, amputations, and trephining (removal of a disc of skull bone). Yet, by the late Eighteenth Century, the scientific basis of surgical techniques was beginning to advance,[10] and American surgical pioneers had performed successful abdominal operations. As early as 1752, Dr. John Bard of New York removed an infected, intra-abdominal pregnancy from a twenty-eight-year-old who made a good recovery. Additional American reports of successful abdominal operations were recorded in the years right after the revolution.[11]

How wounds healed had captured Jones's interest as a medical student, and in 1776, the process of wound healing was still a puzzle for him and his contemporaries. Suppuration from infection was so common that most physicians through history, even going back to the great Greek physicians Hippocrates of Kos (460-375 BCE) and Galen of Pergamon (129-199 AD), thought it was part of normal healing. In his text, Jones wrote of wound healing, that "about the fourth day, sooner or later, according to the age of the patient and the heat of the weather, a white ... equal matter called pus appears, is generated in the wound; and this produces happy effects by separating the lacerated vessels and extravasated fluids from the sound parts which then grow up a-fresh,—Hence laudable pus is esteemed by Surgeons the best of signs".[12]

Surgeons at the time were amiss on the cause of inflammation. Jones wrote that "irritation and pain ... are at all times its [inflammation's] immediate or proximate causes; and that, in most cases, if we can prevent pain, we shall proportionately prevent or at least lessen the succeeding symptoms. This is to be done only by the immediate exhibition of sudorific [a medication that induces sweating] anodynes ... bleeding, gentle laxatives, warm baths, and soft cataplasms to the parts affected." He added that controlling pain with opium was essential, and without it, other treatments "will seldom avail". That pus was made up of bacteria, debris, and white blood cells attracted to fight infection and that inflammation was the body's response to invading germs were concepts still almost a century in the future. Similarly, use of handwashing to prevent infection was not yet thought of, and only a few surgeons had begun preliminary experiments with antiseptics.[13]

The greatest barrier to the advance of surgery was how to effectively control pain. At the time of the revolution, the only answer was forcible restraint of the patient and alcohol or opiates. However, because these were only marginally effective, operations were, of necessity, short and simple.[14] The problems surrounding post-operative pain continue to present a challenge to medical treatment of veterans even in the Twenty-First Century.

---

[1] Abigail D. Griesemer et al., "John Jones, MD: Pioneer, Patriot, and Founder of American Surgery," *World Journal of Surgery* 34, no. 4 (April 2010): 605-609.

[2] Griesemer et al., "John Jones, MD,"

[3] Ibid.

[4] Ibid.

[5] Editorial JAMA 1964.

[6] John Jones, Plain Concise Practical Remarks, on the Treatment of Wounds and Fractures (Philadelphia: Robert Bell, 1776), 1.

[7] Jones, Plain Concise Practical Remarks, cover page.

[8] Jones, 5-6.

[9] Jones, 10-11.

[10] Early European physiologists had been uncovering how the body worked for almost two hundred years. William Harvey of England first described human circulation in 1618, and physicians in Europe and North America learned anatomy by dissecting human cadavers. Practicing new techniques, innovative surgeons were developing techniques for removal of breast and tongue cancers, cutting out bladder and kidney stones, and even removing cataracts of the eye, but surgery in the abdomen and chest was still rare. Among the great innovators and teachers was the French

Notes, continued

surgeon Jean Louis Petit (1674-1750), who developed the tourniquet to stop bleeding during an amputation and techniques for mastectomy for breast cancer including removal of the lymph nodes—setting the practice that would persist into modern times (Sheldon, 14, 17). In the British Isles, the master surgeon John Hunter (1728-1793) had extraordinary influence, extending to the Americas through his students. Born in rural Scotland as the tenth and youngest child in the family, he learned medicine and surgery in London in the 1740s and 1750s. His ten-year older brother William, also well known as a physician, obstetrician, and anatomist, mentored John early in his career. During the Seven Years War, John Hunter served as a British Army surgeon when he developed his interest in wounds and their care. After that war, Hunter returned to London to start his own anatomy school and practice. Like many geniuses, he could be abrasive, adversarial, and eccentric. He had a temper but also a sense of humor and good wit (Sheldon,14). His legacy was his myriad contributions and his students. Hunter's giant scientific work laid the groundwork in vascular surgery, trauma surgery, burns, and inflammation (Sheldon,17). Hunter developed techniques for treating war wounds and ligating (tying off) an aneurysm of the main artery to the leg. He taught more than forty students, including Americans who would play central roles in the American Revolution: Samuel Bard and John Jones of New York and John Morgan, William Shippen and Benjamin Rush of Philadelphia. Suffering from angina much of his life, Hunter collapsed in a fit of temper and died in October 1793.

[11] Hasselgren, Revolutionary Surgeons.

[12] Jones, Plain Concise Practical Remarks, 16.

[13] The simple intervention of handwashing required knowledge of the germ theory of disease, a development in mid-Nineteenth Century Europe. Indeed, the scientific contributions of the French chemist and microbiologist Louis Pasteur (1822-1895) to understanding germs and disease had such impact that his name has become a household word. Hence, we use the term "pasteurization" to kill harmful bacteria in milk and food. The complementary development of handwashing was the brainchild of a young Hungarian obstetrician, Ignaz Phillipp Semmelweis, who worked in the world-famous Vienna General Hospital in the 1840s. Semmelweis keenly deduced that outbreaks of fever in maternity wards were spread by physicians who did bare-handed obstetrical examinations shortly after performing ungloved autopsies on corpses of infected women. His intervention of handwashing in basins of chlorinated lime water before the obstetrical examinations was lifesaving. But in very conservative Vienna, the senior medical staff derided Semmelweis. They rejected his concept that doctors could be the vectors of disease. It took a dozen years for Semmelweis to publish his book on the cause of childbed fever and for the absolute correctness of his observations to be recognized. Today,

Notes, continued

Semmelweis is hailed for the introduction of handwashing in the prevention of disease and is recognized as the "Father of Epidemiology." While the discovery of germs was also decades away, some physicians in the Eighteenth Century began looking for antiseptics. In the 1750s, Sir John Pringle, used the term "antiseptic" in his experiments to prevent decay in flesh of killed animals. Across the English Channel, French surgeons discussed use of turpentine, alcohol, benzoin, and aloe. However, wide-spread use of antiseptics for surgery awaited the pioneering work of Scottish physician Joseph Lister with carbolic acid (phenol) in the 1860s.

[14] Ether (chemically, diethyl ether) was first anesthetic (Chang). Although it had been prepared in 1540 by a Prussian botanist, named Valerius Cordus, it took another three hundred years for it be ushered in for pain control during surgery. Initially, ether was used as a recreational drug in England and the United States. American students had "ether frolics" achieving a euphoric feeling by drinking an ounce of liquid ether. The first use of ether as an anesthetic was not until 1842 when Doctor Crawford W. Long of Georgia used it during removal of a neck tumor. But Long did not publish his observation until 1849, and credit for first use of ether is generally attributed to William T. G. Morton, a dentist from Boston. Before Dr. Morton used either, he had attended a demonstration of nitrous oxide (commonly called "laughing gas") for a wisdom tooth extraction by Dr. Horace Wells, also a dentist. Because the demonstration resulted in only partial pain relief, it was considered a failure, setting back the use of nitrous oxide gas as an anesthetic for several years. Morton became very interested, and with Charles Jackson, a Harvard Medical School Professor of Chemistry, he advanced the use of ether. They reasoned that ether had special advantages compared with nitrous oxide. As a liquid, ether could be easily transported, and it had high volatility, meaning it could be administered by inhalation. Further, it needed to be administered only in low concentrations to achieve surgical level anesthesia. On October 16, 1848, Morton carried out the first public demonstration of ether's use in a surgical amphitheater at Massachusetts General Hospital. That operating room, still open to visitors today, is known as the "Ether Dome." The patient, Mr. Gilbert Abott, underwent successful excision of his neck tumor, under safe, effective ether anesthesia. The medical specialty of anesthesiology was born. Morton's technique used a glass globe containing an ether-soaked sponge and a tube with a mouthpiece through which the patient breathed in the anesthetizing vapors. His simple technique proved effective and reversible but was not without problems. It was accompanied by post-operative nausea and vomiting, and the vapors had explosive flammability. Use of ether became adopted quickly world-wide. Because of its relative safety with careful handling and ease of use, ether remained the standard method of general anesthesia for over a century. Since the 1960s, ether has been replaced by other drugs that avoided ether's problems. Today's inhalation anesthetics have a wide margin of safety and are administered via a tube in

Notes, continued

the trachea by complex machines which allow the anesthesiologist to precisely adjust the mix of gas and oxygen. Modern techniques also avoid the potential problem of aspiration of stomach contents into the airway (Chang).

CHAPTER SIX

DR. JOHN JONES HEADS OFF TO WAR, 1777

Following the British conquest of New York City in September 1776, the King's College medical school had to close. Some of the faculty were loyalists, but, as mentioned in Chapter Five, John Jones had openly supported independence for the colonies. Motivated by his patriotic spirit for the cause, Dr. Jones, now one of the most prominent surgeons in the colonies, decided to enlist in the Continental Army. Although his roots were in New York, he travelled to Boston, where in early 1777 a new regiment—the 10th Massachusetts—was being formed with Colonel Thomas Marshall as its commander. The new unit which would have eight companies, together totaling about 600 to 800 soldiers, recruited men from seven counties in Massachusetts and one in New Hampshire. After its formation and training, the regiment was ordered to the Northern Department to fight the invading enemy army from Canada, under British Major General Burgoyne[1].

Dr. Jones's Regimental Hospital

The Tenth Massachusetts was extremely fortunate to have so qualified a surgeon as John Jones. During the war, each regiment had its own surgeon, who owed his loyalty solely to his commanding colonel. There were no requirements for being selected by a colonel as the regimental surgeon, and many surgeons were poorly qualified. The American system was modeled on the British Army, in which the surgeon's station was a lowly one. British regimental surgeons were placed in readiness reports below the ensigns (the lowest ranking officers).[2]

While the Tenth Massachusetts Regiment was in Boston, Dr. Jones would likely have established a regimental hospital to care for the soldiers afflicted with marked cases of wintertime respiratory illnesses or with dysentery or typhus common in crowded conditions. In his book, Jones had already given other surgeons directions about organizing their regimental hospitals. He knew of the hospital's dangers and recommended that "the buildings appropriated to such purposes, should be the most spacious that can be found; for which reason, churches, barns, and every kind of large out-houses, are preferable to close private dwellings; for as the greatest danger arises from foul air".[3] Jones further knew of the consequences of overcrowding and provided his best rule: "admit so few patients into each ward, that a person unacquainted with the danger of bad air, might imagine there was room to take in triple the number". Lastly, he recommended "the utmost possible cleanliness." He thought it necessary to state that the "discharges and dressings [of the sick] should be removed immediately out of the wards; and the floors, after being properly cleaned, may be sprinkled with vinegar''.

Dr. Jones undoubtedly was assisted by one or more surgeon's mates who helped at surgery, distributed medications, and provided other supervised care. Again, following the British medical model, the surgeon's mates' appointments were solely in the hands of the regiment's commanding officer. With no regulations for these appointments, one contemporary British surgeon wrote that he "could point out cases, where a common soldier from the ranks, after assisting the surgeon of the regiment, in spreading plasters for some time ... was appointed mate thereof".[4] To assist the American regimental surgeon and mates, there were also orderlies (men from the ranks assigned to the hospital) and camp followers to provide cleaning, laundering, and some elementary nursing care. With no apothecary on his staff, the American regimental surgeon was dependent upon his own means or the general hospital for medications and supplies, but getting these materials was an ongoing source of conflict between the doctors in the general hospitals and the regimental surgeons.[5]

During disease outbreaks or after a battle, the regimental hospital could quickly become inundated setting the stage for infection spread, and after a battle, the number of wounded could overwhelm the regiment's surgeon and his mates. In these situations, cases were referred to the general hospitals, but the capacity of these higher-level facilities often also became inadequate.[6]

The British invasion from Canada

As introduced in Chapter Three, the British intended to crush the American rebellion in 1777 with a two-pronged strategy. While the main British Army under General Howe was on route to capture Philadelphia, another British Army under General John Burgoyne was authorized from London by the Secretary of State for Colonies to attack from Canada into Upstate New York. The campaign culminated at Saratoga, New York.

Surgeon Jones at Saratoga

Dr. Jones's 10th Massachusetts Regiment was in the thick of battle against the invading British army at Saratoga. His book, written before 1777, does not include what it was like to be a regimental surgeon on the battlefield, but other sources help to form a picture.

At Saratoga, the Americans picked their defensive position first and awaited the advance of the Crown's forces. In preparation for battle, Dr. Jones would have set up his regimental hospital in a tent 300 to 500 yards behind the infantry, in a protected spot, if possible, such as behind a hill. Battlefield scenes were filled with agony and horror, made even worse when victorious troops looted the enemy wounded. Wounded men were cared for during or after the battle either right on the field by a surgeon's mate or were taken to the regimental hospital, but there was no organized system for getting the wounded to a surgeon.[7] More fortunate wounded might be transported quickly to the regimental hospital with a stretcher, cart, wheelbarrow, or sling, but often the wounded remained on the field in pain and bleeding, even overnight.[8] When a regiment was hard hit, the surgeon had no hope of caring for all his regiment's casualties right away. Hurriedly, even a veteran surgeon like Dr. Jones and his mates might be able to merely dress most wounds or give pain medications while prioritizing surgery for men with hemorrhaging wounds. Inundated by the incoming wounded, the regimental surgeon might refer high-ranking wounded officers, complicated cases, or simply those too numerous for him to handle to the general hospital. Most wounds became infected owing to the conditions in the field and the lack of sterile technique in care. For long term care of wounded such as men with protracted infection, the American Army established large convalescent hospitals, located typically in a safe area, many miles from the battlefront. During the war, there were as many as nineteen of these hospitals in locations from Rhode Island to Virginia.[9]

Weaponry and Tactics

The battle wounds that Dr. Jones cared for must be understood in the context of Eighteenth-Century weaponry and tactics and of the war itself.[10] Armies of the Eighteenth Century consisted of the infantry, artillery and cavalry. In the British Army, infantrymen were organized in Regiments of Foot, generally about 800 men. Washington organized his infantry along British lines, but regiment size was more variable.

Muskets and rifled weapons had different advantages for the fighting soldier. Rifled weapons gave the ball a spin, leading to greater range and accuracy, but were slower to load. The standard weapon for the British infantryman was a smooth bore, muzzle loading musket, commonly called the "Brown Bess". It was of 0.75 caliber and had the old flintlock firing mechanism, making it unreliable particularly in damp or wet weather. An infantry man needed two opposing teeth to bite off the paper end of the cartridge. He then emptied the one hundred grains of black powder into the muzzle and rammed the paper wadding and finally the one-ounce lead ball down the steel barrel. The men were drilled to fire three shots a minute. Pointing the Brown Bess forward but not really aiming, on command, the infantry man squeezed the trigger. The flint hit the steel plate of the flintlock, sending sparks into the gunpowder and igniting the charges. The force of the explosions in the musket's breech accelerated the ball across the field at one thousand feet per second. The mass firing from hundreds of muskets was designed to have a devastating effect. The musket was usually fitted with a lock to fix a seventeen-inch-long, steel bayonet.

The American Army used the Brown Bess musket, the French Charleville Musket, or sometimes home-made weapons. Infantry tactics were dictated by the musket's features. The greater accuracy and longer range of rifled weapons were accompanied by slower loading, about one shot per minute. In the American Army, rifled weapons were not used by regular infantry and were reserved mainly for scouts and some militia units. The British Army used the standard Brown Bess musket for infantry units. Specialized British units such as rangers and scouts may have used rifled weapons.

The medical consequences of a wound from a musket or a rifled weapon differed. The lead ball fired from the smooth bore musket had lower velocity and caused less damage than the higher velocity ball fired from a rifle.[11]

Field artillery fired three, six, or eighteen pound shot which could be solid ball, grapeshot (a tightly packed canvas bag of small iron or lead shot), or canister (a closed metal casing filled with small shot). The latter two were used against charging infantry. Larger cannon and mortars (which fired in a high lobbing arc) were often used in siege warfare. Artillery supported infantry but did not have the destructive power of weapons developed in later times for use in the American Civil War (1861-1865).

Cavalry units in the Revolutionary War were small and used for scouting, raiding, and supporting infantry in battle. They could be used to attack an enemy line in the flank or chase down fleeing infantry. Cavalrymen were armed with pistols, sabers, and carbines (short-barreled muskets). Dragoon units were mounted infantry who carried carbines.

In the Eighteenth Century, European amies mainly followed the tactic of two forces facing each other in linear array, usually two or three ranks deep. The men marched shoulder to shoulder when advancing toward an enemy infantry line but would spread out to a few feet apart if facing cannon fire. When the enemy lines were within range of about fifty to seventy-five yards, the lines halted, presented arms, and fired their muskets. Because of the musket's inaccuracy, its effectiveness depended upon its mass firing effect. Due to the explosions of powder and clouds of white smoke from mass firing, it was hard to see or hear commands in battle. Drums beat out the orders. After the first volley fire, the infantry reloaded and fired one or more volleys. When one side seemed to gain the advantage, it would be ordered to close on the enemy, with deadly bayonets bristling from its front. Fierce hand-to-hand combat was fought with bayonets, swords, and musket butts. To prepare for these scenes of horror and fear, infantrymen were drilled to develop discipline and steadiness under fire. Particularly in the British Army, its veteran regiments struck fear in the enemy by their loud thumping drums and fearsome scarlet lines.

To attack a well-defended position, the approaching army might use siege tactics to block food, supplies and reinforcements. Then, using a series of trenches, the attacking army brought its cannon and soldiers closer to the defenders' walls. Through bombardment and direct assault, the attacking force expected to eventually achieve victory. The American culminating victory at Yorktown (October 1781) resulted from the successful Franco-American siege.

For warfare in North America, both the British and American Armies developed new tactics which they used in selected circumstances. Americans, familiar with hunting in the woods, naturally adopted hit and run maneuvers and the ambush as in attacking the British retreating from Concord (April 1775). For fighting in the North American wilderness, the British Army developed light infantry for quick maneuvering, ranger units for scouting, and flank companies to counter ambushes.

The American Army often prepared defensive positions with spade and shovel work and awaited the British to attack them. The Battles of Bunker Hill (1775), Brooklyn (1776), White Plains (1776), Brandywine (1777), and Guilford Court House (1781) all followed this tactic.

Based upon the weaponry and tactics, it is not surprising that the most common battlefield wounds were musket ball shots, stabbings from bayonets, and slashings and cuttings from sabers and swords. Though cannon ball wounds maimed horribly or killed instantly, they were less frequent mainly due to fewer of these weapons, and slower firing.

Dr. Jones in surgery

When Dr. Jones enlisted, he likely brought his own instruments with him. These probably included probes, bullet forceps, catheters, lancets, ivory and pewter syringes, tourniquets, crooked needles, straight needles, scissors, retractors, scalpels, trepanning instruments, and amputating instruments (curved amputation knives, straight amputation knives, and amputation saws). For use in surgery, the Medical Department authorized full medical chests for surgeons who did not have their own instruments and to provide an assortment of sponges, twine, tape, splints, pins, compresses, bandages, flannel, sutures of linen, cotton or silk, lint, and rags. However, because nearly all the instruments had to be imported, they were, like medications, often in short supply in North America.

We may imagine the senior regimental surgeon, Dr. John Jones, in his hospital tent on September 19, 1777. As the fighting rages that afternoon a few hundred yards away at Freeman's Farm, two orderlies bring a young lieutenant to the hospital in a cart. The lieutenant's right arm is soaking the bandages with blood. He is ashen with a glassy look in his blue eyes. With a nod of his head, Dr. Jones directs the orderlies to the empty operating table in the back of the tent. The table has been fashioned from a spare dresser that Colonel Marshall donated to the hospital. To soften its surface, the mate has covered it with two blankets, but both are spotted with dried blood from previous cases. Dr. Jones's instruments are set out in their velvet-lined kit. These too are speckled with blood as washing them thoroughly was not yet appreciated as part of infection prevention. The veteran surgeon strides to the lieutenant's side. Jones gently examines his arm and decides that it is so shattered from a cannonball that immediate amputation is needed.[12] Knowing that the wounded officer is just barely conscious, the great surgeon nevertheless consoles him, offering empathic words about the quickness of the operation, the use of opiates, and the chances for survival. The lieutenant is strapped with large leather belts into position for easy surgical access on the make-shift operating table, and laudanum is administered orally to quickly induce a half sleep.

Dr. Jones has washed his hands quickly to remove the slippery blood from his previous case. Yet dried blood persists around his fingernails, and his operating apron is soiled and spattered. Germs that cause post-operative infection remain under his nails and in his apron. At the table, across from Jones, there is his trusty surgeon's mate, and two burly fellows, one on each side, who are needed to restrain the patient, despite the leather straps. For the lieutenant, through his pain and opiate-induced semiconsciousness, the scene is hardly comforting as soldiers recovering from other operations are nearby, moaning or crying out, and as already amputated limbs pile up. In the distance, the horrid sounds of on-going battle add to the soldier's fear.

The surgeon's mate applies a leather tourniquet to the officer's arm a few finger breadths above the incision site. With his large, curved knife, the surgeon deftly makes a circumferential incision through the skin of the patient's arm, three inches above the wound. The patient writhes and hauntingly cries out for a few seconds. Jones concentrates on his work and avoids thinking about the young officer's agony. To minimize the pain, he must finish the case quickly. The surgeon's mate retracts the skin flap so that the surgeon may incise the tendon and muscles. With a small circular knife, the surgeon swiftly cuts through these tissues down to the bone. With his bare hands, the mate retracts the stubs of the muscles while the surgeon reaches for the bone saw. It takes only a few seconds to cut through the humerus bone, an inch in diameter. The amputated arm is placed in a basket to be buried later that day along with sawed off limbs from other cases. Even with the tourniquet tightly in place, blood still spurts from the brachial artery supplying the arm. The surgeon swiftly controls the hemorrhage by clamping and tying off the blood vessel. Releasing the tourniquet, the surgeon sees a few bleeding veins and ligates them too. Then, when satisfied that he had stanched the hemorrhage, the surgeon pulls the skin flap down over the stump of bone and muscle and quickly sutures it closed with a needle attached to heavy silk thread.

The surgeon's mate dresses the stump with thick cotton bandages and wraps it tightly. The surgeon rinses his hands once more of the sticky, partially dried blood in a tableside basin and gets ready for his next case. He has done hundreds of amputations, and this one took just sixty seconds. There is no time to rest as he looks from the tent to see two men bearing another wounded soldier on a stretcher.

For the young lieutenant, his ordeal continues post-operatively with pain only partially controlled by opiates and with infection developing at the surgical site.[13] The findings of infection—increasing pain, fever, swelling, and redness—begin a few days after surgery. The lieutenant has been strong and healthy, but over the next few days, the stump becomes more painful, hot, and reddened. By six days after the amputation, pus begins to ooze between the stitches. Dr. Jones has expected to see this as it occurs after nearly every amputation. Two days later, the sutured stump bursts open discharging copious amounts of foul, yellow gray pus. Dr. Jones responds by letting more blood. He knows that healing will take months and arranges for the lieutenant to be transferred to the convalescent hospital nearest his home. Jones hopes the junior officer will make it there and eventually to home.

There's no vacant table in Dr. Jones's tent as the orderlies bring in a stretcher bearing a wounded private and place it on the earthen floor.[14] Because of continuous bleeding, the orderly had to bandage the soldier's thigh while they were still on the battlefield. The private is alert and bravely tells Dr. Jones that he was at Freeman's Farm when he was wounded in the afternoon's fighting. Jones kneels beside the young private and gives him a vial of laudanum to help with the pain. The surgeon then inspects the wound. It is badly contused, a mix of lacerated, bluish-black tissue, with bright red bleeding. As his assistants restrain the soldier, Jones cuts away the blackened skin and muscle with his scalpel and tissue forceps and then dilates the entry wound. The private writhes in pain and screams out.

Working facilely, Jones explores the wound with his bare index finger. The prevailing surgical thinking is to remove the ball for fear that leaving it leads to deadly infection.[15] Jones feels the ball at the tip of his finger. He successfully passes a narrow bullet forceps along the track, grasps the ball, and extracts it gently. To his surgeon's mate, he explains how fortunate this soldier is. Musket balls, he explains, have a nasty habit of spinning after entry and ricocheting after striking bone, sometimes taking maddening courses in the body or becoming firmly lodged in bone. From his vast experience, Surgeon John Jones subscribes to the dictum that "we ought not to attempt the extraction of anything which lies beyond the reach of the finger".[16] Jones takes a deep breath and sees a small vessel spurting bright red blood, signifying an arterial laceration. Again, he isolates the artery, clamps it with his fine instrument, and ties it off with a cotton suture to prevent ongoing hemorrhage.

To conclude the surgery, Jones removes several fragments of fractured bone and bits of uniform that had been drawn into the wound. With his curved needle, he then places three sutures to control the superficial bleeding, and the surgeon's mate dresses the wound with layers of clean bandages. For care after all gunshot wounds, Jones takes "as much blood as his strength will bear." He uses "repeated bleedings ... [as] they generally prevent and always lessen the fever and inflammation" plus mild laxatives and the "almost divine power of opium".[17]

If a soldier were wounded in the head, Dr. Jones would have likely performed trephining, surgical removal of a disc of skull bone to relieve developing pressure on the brain. The surgical instrument, called a trephine, had a bone or steel handle which was affixed to a three-inch long steel shaft. At the other end was a cylindrical saw, three-fourths of an inch in diameter. Dr. Jones would have placed the teeth of the trephine against the skull and circumscribed a disc with twisting pressure. With forceps, he would remove the disc of bone from the skull and fill the trepanned hole with lint. Outcomes were nearly always poor owing primarily to the underlying injury but also to the likely onset of brain infection. (See Appendix B for details.)

For stabbing and cutting wounds from bayonets or swords, Dr. Jones's treatment would have depended upon the depth and location. Superficial cutting or slashing wounds would have been treated by closure with sutures or with sticking plasters. Deep, penetrating wounds of an extremity would be dilated and bandaged. If an abscess developed, it required drainage. If gangrene set in, an amputation was in order. Most bayonet and sword wounds entering the chest or abdominal cavity were fatal, either immediately from hemorrhage or after a few days from infection, organ injury, pneumonia, peritonitis and shock.

Fractures occurred commonly among the soldiers from hand-to-hand combat or from falls. With a simple fracture of a limb, Dr. Jones would have reduced the broken bones "as nearly as possible to their natural situation, and ... retain[ed] them there, by the most easy, simple, and effectual means".[18] Most commonly, this was performed by two assistants applying traction and counter-traction "with more or less violence ... until the extremities of the broken bone were brought opposite to each other when the Surgeon finishes the coaptation or setting." The limb was immobilized by a splint or by an eighteen-tailed bandage, the tails of which were overlapped obliquely to provide as much tightness as needed.[19] Dr. Jones treated complicated fractures by amputation. These complications included joint involvement, abscess or gangrene, shattered limbs, or severe bleeding.

Dr. Jones remained with his regiment through the Saratoga campaign. At the Battles of Saratoga, the American casualties numbered 90 killed and 240 wounded. For the British, the numbers were much worse: 440 killed, 695 wounded, and over 6000 captured. Dr. Jones likely performed several operations on wounded from the Tenth Massachusetts.

Because of poor health and worsening asthma, Dr. Jones moved to Philadelphia where he continued to serve in the army until 1781 at which time he resigned his commission. Late in Doctor Jones's career, he cared for Benjamin Franklin in the sage's last days and notably for George Washington, who as president was suffering from pneumonia. In a twist of fate, the next day, Jones developed symptoms of fever, diarrhea, and fatigue. Washington survived another eight years, but adding to Jones's long-standing asthma, the pneumonia claimed the great surgeon's life five days after he successfully treated Washington.[20]

---

[1] American Revolutionary War Continental Regiments, website.

[2] Hamilton, 3.

[3] Jones, 110-111.

[4] Hamilton, 3.

[5] Reiss, 58, 64-65.

[6] Reiss, 39.

[7] In 1777, Congress authorized the quartermaster to provide wagons with litters to evacuate the wounded, but like so many congressional directives, lack of funding meant few were available. (Reiss, 3).

[8] The Battles at Saratoga in September and October 1777 were American victories fought in the sparsely populated country of upper New York State. Elsewhere in September, the Battle of the Brandywine ended at nightfall, an overwhelming British victory not far from the cities of Wilmington, Delaware and Philadelphia. After that battle, some American wounded were admitted to British military hospitals, and American doctors were permitted to cross lines to care for their own wounded in British hospitals. Doctor Benjamin Rush was allowed to enter the battlefield the next day to treat surviving American wounded still on the field (Reiss,169).

[9] Reiss, 44-45.

[10] American Revolution Facts, website.

[11] In the Eighteenth Century, solid lead balls fired from muskets or pistols had low velocity when wounding a soldier. As a result, the tissue damage was mainly along the bullet's path. There was minimal cavitation (damage to adjacent structures). Bullets from rifles and later weapons had much greater velocity and caused wider tissue destruction. For wounds of the extremities, the prevailing surgical thinking was to remove the ball and other debris drawn into the track to prevent suppuration and death. Whether to persist at efforts to remove the ball was a matter of debate. No less a surgical figure than the famed Scottish surgeon John Hunter (1728-

Notes, continued

1793) knew that the body sometimes could adapt to the foreign body and that a bullet might work its way to the surface. Accordingly, he advocated avoiding probing and removing bullets except in a few circumstances such as when gangrene developed or when a ball pressed on a vital spot. As exemplified in the illustrative case, Jones's opinion was an intermediate one. Remove the ball if easily done; otherwise, leave it. Bullet wounds of the head were often treated by trephining but were usually fatal due to severe brain injury. Wounds in a large joint such as the knee required amputation immediately. When there was a gunshot wound or penetrating wound of the chest or abdomen, injury to vital organs such as the heart and aorta were known to be fatal. Injury to other organs, Jones wrote, including even the lungs, liver, and intestines were "only hazardous in the proportion to the nature of the offices they perform in the animal oeconomy" (Jones, 26). In such cases, though, surgical treatment was limited to dilating the bullet's entry orifice. Open surgery of the abdomen or chest was nearly always out of the question. If the wound involved laceration of the large intestine, for example, the soldier progressed inexorably to peritonitis (infection of the abdominal cavity) and agonizing death. As testimony to Jones's surgical brilliance, he devised a technique for "a complaint of a very singular nature," namely, a musket ball causing a rib fracture by passing in an oblique direction but without entering the chest cavity. Here, Jones observed the consequence from the sharp points of the rib fracture was puncture and collapse of the lung, inducing difficulty in breathing or even "absolute suffocation." Jones's solution for this life-threatening wound was to make a small incision in the chest wall to let the trapped air escape and permit the lung to re-expand. This operation, called then and now "thoracentesis," is used with a modern technique for collapsed lung.

[12] Amputation was feared by soldiers not only because of the agonizing surgical ordeal and risk of dying, but also for the lifetime of limitations for those fortunate enough to survive. For the Eighteenth-Century surgeon, amputation was the most common operation and the solution to many problems: gangrene, abscess of a joint, gunshot wounds of a large joint, or, as in this case, a shattered limb. Yet many soldiers thought they would rather die than be maimed, due to not wishing to become a burden on families needing able-bodied men to do farmwork or other labor.

[13] When infection complicated an amputation, there were three possible outcomes. First, in up to half or more of cases, uncontrolled infection (called "cellulitis") spread up the arm or leg and throughout the body, leading to organ failure, shock and death. In terms of modern microbiology, this outcome was likely caused by the bacterium, Streptococcus pyogenes, also called Group A streptococci, which today causes "strep throat" and "the flesh eating" disease. Second, in some cases, the soldier's immune (infection-fighting) system controlled and localized the infection, leading to an abscess. Abscesses were mainly caused by the bacterium, Staphylococcus aureus, still a common cause of community- and hospital-

Notes, continued

acquired infections. When an abscess developed, it sometimes burst open spontaneously. If not, the surgeon waited for just the right time for the abscess to come to a head and then lanced (in medical terms, "incised and drained") the abscess. It often took repeated drainage procedures and weeks to months to heal large abscesses. Even then, in some cases, death followed from protracted infection. Third, in a minority of cases, the infection healed without complications over many weeks. During post-operative infections, the surgeon and his staff administered well-intentioned treatments of the day: bleedings, purges, leeches, and blistering plasters.

[14] In modern warfare, American forces have highly effective "triage" systems in which a wounded soldier is first evacuated to a field aid station. Those with minor wounds are treated there while those with more serious injuries are transported quickly to full-service hospitals.

[15] As a historical note, the practice of removing the ball continued well into the Nineteenth Century. Indeed, Candice Millard in *Destiny of the Republic* makes the case that after President James Garfield's chest wound in 1881 by an assassin, his doctors brought on his death by excessive attempts to remove the ball (Millard). In current practice, the decision to remove or observe a bullet is a complex one depending upon its location, the wounded patient's status, and the velocity of the bullet. For example, a bullet by the spine is removed because it may cause neurologic injury while a bullet deep in muscle may be observed rather than removed.

[16] Jones, 91.

[17] Jones, 94.

[18] Jones, 31.

[19] Jones, 38; Wilbur, 35.

[20] Griesemer.

Chapter Seven

Dr. Albigence Waldo Endures Hardships at Valley Forge, 1777-1778

Albigence Waldo had a perspective like that of no other Revolutionary War doctor. As a surgeon in the First Connecticut Regiment, he wrote in his diary and letters home about the sick and the lame, but what makes him unique is his account of the human side of soldiering. Waldo held nothing back. He revealed his longings for family, anger about poor food, criticism of "Country Gentlemen," hardships endured from the bitter cold, and complaints about his own illnesses. But he also wrote glowingly of his admiration for Washington and about respect for the "Indians." He was an amateur musician and a devoted poet. His diary is laced with humor, home-spun philosophy, and empathy. And Waldo just happened to serve at the historic winter encampment at Valley Forge.

Waldo was born in 1750 in Pomfret, Connecticut. After receiving his education from the parish minister, he served an apprenticeship in nearby Canterbury. Waldo's timing was serendipitous because the Pomfret town doctor moved to Vermont opening the practice opportunity for him in his hometown.[1] In November 1772, Dr. Waldo married Lydia Hurlbut. Together they had seven children, but when the war broke out, he like so many other young men answered the call. He left his family and practice to join a Connecticut militia company as a clerk. On July 6, 1775, he became a surgeon's mate in the Eighth Connecticut Regiment but was discharged in September because of ill-health. He improved over the next year and in December 1776 he returned to service as chief surgeon on a Connecticut armed ship. Shortly, though, he accepted an invitation from his former Connecticut commander, Col.

Jedidiah Huntington, to join his newly-raised First Connecticut Regiment, now as regimental surgeon.

From Germantown to Valley Forge, 1777

In spring 1777, Waldo and his regiment were stationed at Peekskill, New York, along the lower Hudson River. In September, after the Continental Army's defeat at Brandywine (September 11, 1777), the First Connecticut was ordered to Pennsylvania. Two weeks after the Brandywine, the British captured Philadelphia. Yet Washington was not done and attacked the main British position in Germantown, outside the American capital, on October 4th. Waldo's Connecticut regiment arrived in time for the battle and formed part of the American left flank. The Battle of Germantown started off well for the Americans as their parallel attacking columns made initial progress. Then the attack fell apart. Washington's plan was too complicated. Heavy fog caused delays and confusion, and the main American column got hung up attacking a small British position inside a stone mansion, called the Chew House. The British had time to regroup and then sent the Americans reeling. American losses included 700 killed and wounded and over 400 captured. After two more months of maneuvering, Washington decided to establish a winter encampment. He chose Valley Forge, nineteen miles from the British in Philadelphia. In Valley Forge, Washington expected an adequate supply of food for his 12,000-man army from rich nearby farms, and from surrounding woodlands that would supply plenty of timber to build huts. Washington was sure he could counter any British maneuver that winter or the following spring. All Washington had to do was keep the army intact.

But encampment at Valley Forge proved difficult. From the outset, clothing was in short supply. Of Washington's 12,000 men, 2000 arrived barefoot. Being shoeless was not uncommon particularly among poor, rural peoples and the enslaved, but at Valley Forge, the problem was one of supply, not individual poverty. Shelters had to be built from scratch, and just feeding the army became a Herculean task for nearly the entire winter. Productive farmers preferred the gold offered by British purveyors rather than the nearly worthless Continental currency.[2]

Surgeon Waldo's Diary

On route to Valley Forge, on December 14th, just ahead of winter, Waldo was already weary. His journal entry read,

> The Army which has been surprisingly heathy hitherto, now begins to grow sickly from continued fatigues they have suffered this Campaign. Yet they still show a spirit of Alacrity & Contentment not to be expected from so young Troops. I am Sick—discontented—and out of humour. Poor food—hard lodging—Cold Weather—fatigue—Nasty Cloaths—nasty Cookery—Vomit half my time—smoak'd out of my senses—the Devil's in't—I can't Endure it—Why are we sent here to starve and Freeze—What sweet Felicities have I left at home; A charming Wife—pretty Children—Good Beds—good food—good Cookery—all agreeable—all harmonious. Here all Confusion-smoke & Cold--hunger & filthyness—A pox on my bad luck. There comes a bowl of beef soup—full of burnt leaves and dirt, sickish enough to make a Hector spue—away with it Boys—I'll live like the Chameleon upon Air."[3, 4]

Yet by the next day, his entry reflected his underlying optimistic philosophy. He wrote,

> Mankind are never truly thankfull for the Benefits of life, until they have experience'd the want of them. The Man who has seen misery knows best how to enjoy good. He who is always at ease & has enough of the Blessings of common life is an Impotent Judge of the feelings of the unfortunate.[5]

The army marched into the encampment site on December 19, 1777. Washington and some officers made headquarters at a stone residence, but the rest of the army had to set up their tents. Immediately, they got to building rude huts, each fourteen by sixteen feet and housing twelve men. On December 21st, Waldo complained to his wife in a letter, "Heartily wish myself at home ... my Skin & eyes are almost spoil'd with continual smoke. A general cry thro' the Camp this Evening among the Soldiers, "No Meat! No Meat!"—the Distant vales Echo'd back the melancholly sound—"No Meat! No Meat!" For dinner, they had "Nothing but Fire Cake (a mixture of flour, water and some fat) & Water."[6]

The next day, still in his tent, Waldo was consumed by bitter weather and hunger. He wrote, "... excessive Cold & uncomfortable last Night—my eyes are started out from their Orbits like a Rabbit's eyes, occasion'd by a great Cold & Smoke ... I am ashamed to say it, but I am tempted to steal Fowls if I could find them, or even a whole Hog, for I feel as if I could eat one." On Christmas Day, with hut building going slowly, Dr. Waldo lamented, "the poor Sick, suffer much in Tents this cold Weather."[7]

For men in tents and later in drafty, smokey huts with inefficient, crude fireplaces, the winter weather was harsh. For the month of December 1777, temperatures averaged 32.4 degrees and rose a bit to 35.4 degrees in January and 37.0 degrees in February, but at night the temperature often fell to the low teens or single digits. On December 27th, it was six degrees; on January 15th, twelve degrees. Snow fell heavily on December 27th, January 11th and February 7th.[8] Snow was so deep after the February blizzard that men could not stir from their huts. That winter, the ground was snow-covered for twenty-nine days, and there were many days of soaking, cold rain.

Life was made even more difficult for Waldo by "Country Gentlemen," lobbing criticisms from the comfort of the homes.

In his journal, Waldo defended his commander in chief and the army with great admiration. On December 26th, he wrote:

> Many Country Gentlemen in the interior parts of the States who get wrong information of the Affairs & state of our Camp, are very much Surprized at G Washington's delay to drive off the Enemy, being falsely inform'd that his Army consists of double the Number of the Enemy's—such wrong information serves not to keep up the spirit of the People, as they must be by and by undeceiv'd to their no small disappointment;—it brings blame on his Excellency, who is deserving of the greatest encomiums; it brings disgrace on the Continental Troops, who have never evidenced the least backwardness in doing their duty, but on the contrary, have cheerfully endur'd a long and very fatigueing Campaign.[9]

At year's end, Waldo's optimism broke through. On New Year's Eve, "We got some Spirits and finish'd the Year with a good Drink & thankfull hearts in our new Hutt, which stands on an Eminence that overlooks the Brigade, & in sight of the Front Line." His buoyant entry on January 1,1778 began, "I am alive." By now, many of the huts were close to completion giving the encampment the appearance of "a spacious City." Indeed, with 12,000 troops, Valley Forge was the third largest "city" in North America after Philadelphia and New York. It had a larger population than either Boston or Charleston.

On New Year's Day, Waldo reflected tenderly about his friends, their suffering, their gratification, and their cause. "Nothing tends to the establishment of the firmest Friendship like Mutual Sufferings which produces mutual Intentions and endeavours for mutual Relief which in such cases are equally shar'd with pleasure and satisfaction—in the course of this, each heart is laid open to full view—the similar passions in each, approximate themselves by a certain impulsive sympathy, which terminates in lasting esteem."[10]

Two days later, he wryly referred to his nearly completed hut as "rather our Hermit's Cell." Then, showing grace while facing adversity, he wrote that after breakfast "with thankful hearts for the little we had, took care of the Sick, according to our dayly practice."[11]

Although Waldo does not specify the diseases of his sick, certainly wintertime respiratory illnesses (including pneumonia and influenza) must have been at the top of the list because of exposure and malnourishment. Skin afflictions were common under these wintry, crowded conditions. On January 8th,1778, Washington noted that too many men were unfit for duty because of "the itch" (mainly scabies, an infestation by a burrowing insect, called a mite). Treatments included an ointment of sulfur in hog's lard. When medical sulfur stocks ran out, doctors sought crude sulfur from the artillery companies.[12] The itch was so intense that individual solders resorted to self-treatment, sometimes with dire results. One soldier smeared his body with a mercury ointment, and another drank one and half pints of rum. They both died. With smallpox inoculations in the army widely used since February 1777 (see Chapter Two), mortality from that disease was low, but many men had generally mild, post-inoculation cases, which lasted nevertheless two to three weeks. In March, the number was reported to be 3,000. As the winter dragged on, the huge encampment grew foul. During a visit, Dr. Benjamin Rush found the camp "dirty and stinking, the men filthy and ragged." General Anthony Wayne called the whole army sick and crawling with vermin.[13] These conditions set the stage for the familiar afflictions of dysentery and typhus.

In keeping with his humanity and empathy for the enlisted men, Dr. Waldo was also ahead of his times, an advocate for respect and equality for an "Indian." He was called to see an ill soldier "tho't to be dying—he expir'd before I reach'd the Hutt. He was an Indian—an excellent Soldier—and an obedient good natur'd fellow." Waldo reasoned, "He engaged for money doubtless as others do;—but he has serv'd his country faithfully—he has fought for those very people who disinherited his forefathers—having finished his pilgrimage, he was discharged from the War of Life & Death. His memory ought to be respected, more than those rich ones who supply the world with nothing better than Money and Vice".[14]

Waldo concludes the entry trenchantly, writing "What a frail-dying creature is Man. We are Certainly not made for this world—daily evidences demonstrate the contrary."[15]

In one of his last entries, dated January 6, Surgeon Waldo demonstrates his humility and love of family.

> — If I should happen to lose this little Journal, any fool may laugh that finds it,—since I know that there is nothing in it but the natural flowings & reflections of my own heart, which is human as well as other Peoples—and if there is a great deal of folly in it—there is no intended Ill nature—and am sure there is much Sincerity, especially when I mention my family, whom I cannot help saying and am not asham'd to say that I Love.[16]

On January 8th, 1778, Waldo received an unexpected furlough and left Valley Forge for home. He soon resumed his service as a regimental surgeon. One of his poems sings humorously of soldiers' camaraderie.

Now Phoebus plunges in the sea
And the gray ev'ning shuts the day,
All parties to prepare for musings
Repair to huts and drink the loosings.
There loud talk soon begins
Of who plays best and who most wins.
Of politics, or frothy matter
That sudden raises general clatter.
Then of cowards, fools, rascals, rattles,
Of duels, heroes, wars, and battles,
Of fornicators, witches, scolds,

Fatigues and hardships, heats and colds,
Of beauty, women, wine, and love,
Of thundering armies and of Jove.
Huzza! The chorus loudly cry,
Responsive vales *Huzza!* reply.
Toasts for the Cause, for sweethearts, wives,
Long peace, long health, and happy lives.[17]

While Waldo was in the service, his family fell on hard times economically. Pay in the Continental Army was paltry. In 1778, an infantryman received less than seven dollars per month, a captain forty dollars per month, and a colonel seventy-five dollars per month. Hospital and regimental surgeons received about forty dollars per month.[18]

Waldo was furloughed from Valley Forge in January 1778 and served until he resigned in October 1779 to return to his practice in Pomfret. There, he developed a wide reputation as a skilled surgeon. His first wife Lydia died in 1785. Waldo then married Lucy Cargill, with whom he had two more children. Waldo died in 1794, a month before his forty-fourth birthday.

The inscription on his graveside monument reads in part:

To the Memory
Of ALBIGENCE WALDO, Surgeon,
Who, attentively studying the Works of God
In the admirable frame of Man,
Rose to eminent distinction
In the noble art of healing;
His name was Charity
His actions, Humanity;
His intercourse with men, benevolence & love.[19]

Afterwards at Valley Forge

After Waldo left Valley Forge in January 1778, there remained still over two months of harsh winter. In early February, almost four thousand Valley Forge soldiers were unfit for duty, mainly because of "scarcity of clothing" and exposure.[20]

To care for the sick, general hospitals were set up not far away at Reading, Bethlehem, Easton, Lititz, and Yellow Springs. The village of Yellow Springs, located ten miles west of Valley Forge, was already considered a health resort for its natural springs and baths which were on the farm owned by Dr. Samuel Kennedy. To support the sick and wounded, Dr. Kennedy established hospitals in three barns. Invalids were packed into these hospitals, creating perfect conditions for contagion. Disease was so widespread that Dr. Kennedy fell ill himself and died of putrid fever (typhus).[21] At the Reading hospital (fifty miles from the camp), with a capacity of 360, there were 900 invalids.[22]

Because of the growing numbers of invalids, these makeshift hospitals were insufficient. The Medical Department needed a central facility. Washington chose Yellow Springs. In February, he ordered the construction of a "commodious building ... to serve both as the Yellow Springs Medical Department headquarters and the principal hospital for the camp".[23] Later called Washington Hall, it was large indeed, measuring 106 feet long by 36 feet wide with three full stories plus an attic. On the second floor, there were two large wards, and on the third, there were many small rooms intended, no doubt, for isolation if needed.

Medical illnesses overcame exposure as the major problems in the spring. On April 26, there were "at least one thousand under inoculation for smallpox," and the next day a hospital physician wrote, "Putrid fevers [typhus] abound greatly."[24] To make matters still worse, medical supplies were unreliable. The Apothecary General wrote on May 1, 1778, "We have many important medicines but by no means an assortment sufficient for the army.... We are destitute of almost everything necessary for regimental chests."[25] Even as late as May 1780, 4000 were reported as sick. On May 17th, General Washington visited the Yellow Springs hospitals. "He spoke to every person in their bunks, which exceedingly pleased the sick."[26] By the time the army left Valley Forge in June 1778, between 1,800 and 2,000 men had died of disease.[27]

Nonetheless, the Continental Army not only survived the winter at Valley Forge but was transformed, owing to the drills, maneuvers and discipline instilled by the Prussian Baron von Steuben, who had been appointed Lieutenant General in the Continental Army. The Continentals left as a professional army, ready to take on the British Regulars and capable of winning independence.

---

[1] Albigence Waldo: Surgeon, website Price, Washington Crossing Park

[2] Reiss, 195.

[3] Waldo makes an allusion to Shakespeare in "Hamlet" (Act 3, Scene 2). It is based on an old belief that chameleons survived by air alone, not needing food.

[4] Valley Forge, 1777-1778, website, https://archive.org/stream/jstor-20085750/20085750_djvu.txt, Full text of :Valley Forge, 1777-1778. Diary of Surgeon Albigence Waldo, of the Connecticut Line. Accessed 1/17/26.

[5] Ibid. Diary of Surgeon Albigence Waldo, of the Connecticut Line.

[6] Ibid.

[7] Ibid.

[8] Katz, 10.

[9] Diary of Surgeon Albigence Waldo, of the Connecticut Line.

[10] Ibid.

[11] Ibid.

[12] Reiss, 199-200.

[13] Reiss, 195.

[14] Website, https://allthingsliberty.com/2024/05/albigence-waldo-surgeon-soldier-diarist-poet/ - _edn21"

[15] Ibid.

[16] Ibid.

[17] Diary of Surgeon Albigence Waldo, of the Connecticut Line.

[18] Soldier Pay in the American Revolution, website.

Notes, continued

[19] Albigence Waldo: Surgeon, Soldier, Diarist, Poet. Washington Crossing Historic Park, website.

[20] Gibson, 192-193.

[21] Gibson, 196.

[22] Reiss, 197.

[23] Gibson, 196-197.

[24] Gibson, 213-215.

[25] Gibson, 201.

[26] Gibson, 232.

[27] McGready.

CHAPTER EIGHT

DR. BODO OTTO AND NURSE ABIGAIL HARTMAN RICE MINISTER TO SOLDIERS AT YELLOW SPRINGS, 1778-1781

The entire camp was abuzz as the news spread from regiment to regiment. The army had been in Valley Forge fully six months. Now, on Tuesday, June 18th, 1778, General Washington's spies arrived from Philadelphia with intelligence that the British were evacuating the capital! For the past few weeks, Washington's agents had been bringing him news that there was movement afoot for the British. The spies reported in May that the enemy was putting cannons, horses, and heavy baggage on board their ships at the Philadelphia docks. There were rumors in Philadelphia, the spies heard, that the British wanted to consolidate their army in New York in case of a combined Franco-American attack following the establishment of the alliance, signed February 6, 1778. But now Washington had definitive intelligence not only of the evacuation, but also that only some equipment and few British troops would go back to New York by ship. Most of the British force, he learned, would march overland, through New Jersey, when their columns would he strung out over many miles. Washington knew the enemy would be vulnerable and immediately made plans to intercept them. Some American officers expected the Continental Army to re-take the capital before pursuing the British, but Washington's innate aggressiveness was up. Going to Philadelphia would give the British Army too much of a head start. He was going directly after them. After getting the news, the "Commander-in-Chief led his men in their march eastward through Bucks County

[Pennsylvania] across the Delaware at Coryell's Ferry to meet the English."[1]

The Battle of Monmouth

The Continentals caught up with the British Army ten days later, on an unusually hot and humid day at Monmouth Court House, New Jersey. Washington placed the initial attack under command of American General Charles Lee, but he "lacked confidence in the ability of the soldiers under his command."[2] Lee failed to press the attack and "ceded the initiative" to the rear guard of the British Army. When Washington arrived at the fighting, he was furious. Immediately relieving Lee, Washington rallied the troops he had in the vanguard units and continued the attack. He "gave time for the rest of the Continental Army to ... join the battle." The fighting under the brutal sun "see-sawed back and forth until" about six o'clock in the evening when the British fell back and slipped "away under cover of darkness and resum[ed] their withdrawal to New York City" the next morning. Washington's hope for a definitive victory "devolved into a potential disaster".[3] His casualties totaled 325. American wounded who required long term care were sent to convalescent hospitals such as Yellow Springs and others in the region. The British killed and wounded numbered 381.

Monmouth was the last major action in the North, where for the next three years the British remained in New York City and the Americans held various posts around the British. Eventually, the British would turn their battle initiatives to the South.

Dr. Otto and Nurse Hartman Rice

When the army left Valley Forge, many senior medical officers followed the army on route to Monmouth. Others went to Philadelphia to continue their work there as Congress was also returning. But many sick and wounded remained in the hospitals at Yellow Springs. The man in charge of their care was a sixty-seven-year-old physician, named Bodo Otto, who had emigrated in 1755 from what is now Germany.[4] Dr. Otto received his medical education at the University of Gottingen before coming to America. His reasons for leaving Europe remain a puzzle. After all, he "enjoyed an enviable position" as a physician and belonged to the Evangelical Lutheran Church, which was officially recognized by the Electorate of Hanover, then ruled by George II of Great Britain. Perhaps he opposed British rule of what he might consider German territory. Perhaps, as a forty-four-year-old, Dr. Otto may have emigrated because of a love of adventure or for economic betterment. Whatever his reasons, he sailed to America and settled in Southeastern Pennsylvania, where there were many German immigrants. He quickly became an established physician and soon a political activist. Dr. Otto opposed the Stamp Act of 1765 and served on the Berks County [Pennsylvania] Committee of Public Safety a council of patriot executives. When the war broke out in 1775, he was appointed by Congress to set up a military hospital for treating smallpox in Trenton, New Jersey. Then, during the campaigns of 1776 and 1777, Dr. Otto was in the thick of the action. He served with Washington's main army at the Battle of Long Island (August 1776). In late December, he was part of the heroic crossing of the Delaware River and the subsequent victory over the German mercenaries fighting for the British (called Hessians) at Trenton the next morning. Dr. Otto "selflessly treat[ed] wounded and dying Hessians" as there were very few American wounded. After the Battle of the Brandywine (September 1777), he set up a hospital to care for the wounded in Trinity Lutheran Church in Reading, Pennsylvania. Based on his training, compassion, skills, and field experience, Dr. Bodo Otto was just the right leader for the Yellow Springs hospitals. There he was assisted by his three sons who were also physicians.

From the beginning of his years as director at Yellow Springs hospitals, Dr. Bodo Otto had his hands full owing to a combination of large numbers of sick and wounded, inadequate funding, and continued shortages of medications and supplies.

During the Valley Forge encampment, 1,300 men were treated at Yellow Springs.[5] The patient load at the new general hospital swelled as other hospitals which had been set up during the encampment closed. In August 1778, the Lititz hospital was abandoned and its patients transferred to Yellow Springs.[6] Other hospitals in the region at Easton and the Brethren House Hospital in Bethlehem had moved their patients to Yellow Springs just before the army marched from Valley Forge.[7] In August 1778, there were 725 sick in the hospitals in the vicinity of Yellow Springs. Another 445 had been discharged, and 124 had died.[8] About a year later, Dr. Otto still had sixty-five soldiers under his care.[9] By early 1780, as patients recovered or died, Dr. Otto wrote to Congress, that Yellow Springs "for some time past, ha[d] been maintained for the reception of those afflicted chiefly with chronic disorders."[10]

He was short of medication, food and supplies. Repeatedly, Otto appealed to Congress. In a letter to "the Committee of Congress for Conducting the Medical Department" in May 1780, he wrote,

> ... our necessary stores for the sick are entirely exhausted. There is no money in the hands of the Commissary to purchase fresh provisions, so the sick have been obliged these several past days to eat salt provisions. There is but six days supply of bread on hand, and the gentlemen who have furnished us that article as well as meat for the past two years now refuse to supply us any longer.[11]

With records from 250 years ago so incomplete, there is no reply available.

Bodo Otto was not alone in ministering to the sick and wounded at Yellow Springs. One remarkable "nurse" was another immigrant from Germany, at the time a thirty-six-year-old mother of thirteen. Abigail Hartman came to America as an eight-year-old with her parents in the summer of 1750.[12] The Hartman family sought a new life in America along with "tens of thousands of German-speaking peoples" most likely because of overpopulation in central Europe and land scarcity. In Rotterdam, Abigail and her family boarded the *Royal Union* packed with 500 other emigrants. During the North Atlantic crossing, the storms were so powerful that the passengers became "convinced that the ship with all aboard is bound to sink," but the *Royal Union* made port safely in Philadelphia on August 15, 1750. The Hartman family set up a farm in nearby Chester County. Seven years later, Abigail, aged sixteen, married a young man in his early twenties named Zachariah Rice. She had her first child two years later and gave birth to a child every year between 1760 and 1774 except for 1766. She would eventually give birth to twenty-one children.

The Hartman and Rice families began to take sides in the political debate over Parliament's repressive acts. In 1774, her father, Johannes Hartman, became a member of the Chester County Committee of Safety. The next year, her brother Peter joined the same committee. As the war unfolded, Peter was appointed captain in the county militia in September 1776 and eventually rose to major. Her husband Zachariah also served in the county militia but did not enlist in the regular army. He felt he could not leave his large family behind during years of service.

Abigail's first visit to the Yellow Springs hospital may have been in 1778 to see her husband who was helping to construct Washington Hall. At first, Abigail did not provide direct care but "came on her errands of mercy, carrying food and delicacies to the sick and wounded." Her trips to Yellow Springs became more frequent, and shortly she assumed nursing care of the soldiers.

At the time of the American Revolution, there were many women in the army encampments. Typically, wives, widows, daughters, or mothers, these "camp followers" stayed with the army because they had no other means of support once the men left home.[13] These women, like Abigail Hartman Rice, provided not only basic care including dressing wounds, bathing patients, distributing medications, and even assisting at surgery, but also gave emotional support as "surrogate mothers, sisters and confidants to [sick and wounded] soldiers far from home."[14] They also freed up soldiers for combat roles. In recognition of the value of nursing care, Congress had approved a request from General Washington in July 1775 to assign one nurse for every ten patients with each nurse being paid a monthly wage of two dollars.[15,16]

But even Abigail Hartman Rice's commitment had its limits. After months of giving care and not receiving the pay the nurses had been promised, Hartman Rice and the other nurses "refused serving any longer." At a time when women were "often considered the physical property of their husbands," the Yellow Springs nurses "raised their voices to demand the money" due them. Dr. Otto took up their banner in a letter to Congress in May 1780. Recognizing the nurses' cause, "Washington and Congress heeded their protest and resolved the issue. By the end of the war, some nurses earned greater pay than enlisted men".[17]

Like many other caregivers of the time, Hartman "paid the ultimate price for her service."[18] At Yellow Springs, she contracted an infection, most likely typhus, from one of the soldiers and developed complications from which she "was never able to fully recover." In 1789, she died at home "still suffering from the disease she contracted years prior." She left behind her husband and their twenty-one children.[19]

The saga at Yellow Springs ended in September 1781 when a congressional committee decided that the hospital should be abandoned. The Director General of the Medical Department, Dr. John Cochran, "strenuously opposed this order"[20] but was not successful. Cochran cited "false economy and lack of appreciation of their need and importance" as the reasons Congress ordered the closing. Dr. Otto was directed to transfer his patients to Philadelphia and to report there "where his services would be most needed."[21] With extraordinary dedication and energy, he served in the army until February 1782 when he finally retired at age seventy years. Otto died in Reading in 1787. In his biography of Dr. Otto, originally published in 1937, Gibson summarizes, "the life of Bodo Otto ... includes the experiences of many unsung patriots.... Conscientious and thorough, Dr. Otto met and solved the problems of his times to the best of his understanding and ability; unafraid and with self-confidence, he frequently changed his plans when proved wrong or he thought better opportunities presented themselves."[22] This modest tribute points up Dr. Otto's courage and his use of what we would call today the scientific method: use of data to inform better practice. A more generous tribute was paid to Dr. Otto by a distinguished Pennsylvania historian, Morton L. Montgomery (1846-1933), who wrote:

> Next to Washington, Gates, Mifflin, Wayne and other leading Generals, Dr. Bodo Otto, of Reading Pa, occupied a prominence and rendered useful service equal to any other man who was engaged in the great cause of the Revolution.[23]

---

[1] Gibson, 234.

[2] Monmouth Battle Facts, American Battlefield Trust. Website.

[3] Ibid.

[4] Dr. Bodo Otto Association, website.

[5] Reiss, 196-197.

[6] Gibson, 203.

[7] Ibid., 207-08.

[8] Ibid., 235.

[9] Ibid.,237.

[10] Ibid., 238.

[11] Ibid.

[12] McGready.

Notes, continued

[13] Healing Heroines, website.

[14] The Unsung Patriots, website.

[15] Army Medicine Facebook Post.

[16] The modern nursing profession did not have its origins until the work of Florence Nightingale, a wealthy British woman who led a group of female nurses to care for soldiers in the Crimea in 1854. Even earlier, some physicians had initiated courses for women interested in nursing. In 1798, Dr. Valentine Seaman gave lectures on maternity care in New York. In the early Nineteenth Century, Dr. Joseph Warrington established a similar program in Philadelphia. During the American Civil War (1861-1865), there were hundreds of thousands of casualties, and about 20,000 women and men provided nursing care. In 1873, the first three nursing educational programs opened, in New York and New England. These three "Nightingale schools" were soon followed by many others. By 1900, there were between 400 and 800 nursing schools in the United States. (American Nursing: An Introduction to the Past, Nursing, History, and Health Care.)

[17] McGready.

[18] Ibid.

[19] A memorial plaque is dedicated to her memory in the bell tower of Washington Memorial Chapel at Valley Forge National Historical Park.

[20] Gibson, 241.

[21] Ibid.

[22] Gibson, 435.

[23] Gibson, 436.

CHAPTER NINE

BRITISH DRS. JOHN HUNTER AND JOHN ROLLO FACE INTERMITTENT FEVER, 1778-1783

In 1778, after the Franco-American Alliance was completed, the American Revolutionary War became internationalized. Britain, which began fighting a campaign in the American South, now also had to defend its military and naval bases in the Caribbean. These bases protected the highly profitable economic interests in sugar, coffee, cotton, indigo and the trans-Atlantic trade in enslaved people. Over the remainder of the war, thousands of British soldiers were sacrificed to ravaging tropical diseases while defending these valuable islands from possible attack from the French, Spanish and Dutch American allies.

In Eighteenth-Century North America and Britain, the main diseases of typhus, smallpox, and dysentery struck the poor more than the wealthy; city dwellers more than country dwellers; and rank and file in the army more than officers. By contrast, in the Caribbean, disease brought death and destruction without regard to station or status. No one was safe. Rampaging disease was devastating especially to troops newly arrived from Europe regardless of the colony. British Army doctors in the West Indies struggled to understand the pattern of tropical diseases so that they might limit illnesses and deaths. Two British physicians even wrote books about their experiences. One was Dr. John Hunter (1754-1809), Superintendent of Military Hospitals in Jamaica.[1] The other notable British physician in the Caribbean was Dr. John Rollo, who served on the island of St. Lucia. Both these Eighteenth-Century British medical detectives studied the tropical diseases and would go on to illustrious careers after the war.

"The other" Dr. John Hunter on Jamaica

John Hunter, who was stationed on Jamaica, was born in Scotland in 1754 and received his MD from the University of Edinburgh in 1775. In a portrait of Hunter as a young man, he has a remarkable mop of wavy hair, piled upon a round, intelligent face.[2] He was appointed physician to the army in 1777 and, by age twenty-seven, sailed to Jamaica as military hospital superintendent. Young Hunter must have stepped ashore in Kingston Harbor with a great sense of foreboding about his task ahead and even his own mortality.

Jamaica had been a Crown colony since 1655 and was central to the sugar trade. At the time, its total population was 200,000, the majority of whom were enslaved persons. Jamaica and the other islands in the West Indies were disease ridden with malaria being the most common threat. Europeans were more susceptible to disease from malaria than were enslaved persons of African origin due to African pre-exposure and partial immunity.

Known in the Eighteenth Century as intermittent, remittent, quotidian, tertian or quartan fever, malaria had been recognized for centuries. The term *malaria* derives from the Latin meaning "bad air" as ancient Romans believed it arose from fumes from swampy ground. This concept persisted through the American Revolution and beyond.

Malaria's clinical picture consists of a sudden attack of intermittent fever occurring daily or every third or fourth day. The attack (called a paroxysm in medical language) follows a dramatic course of a chill, fever, and sweat. The paroxysm's onset includes weakness, headache, and sometimes nausea and vomiting. The chill is dramatic as the patient begins to shiver violently. The teeth chatter, and the shivering may cause the bed to shake. The fever is high, even up to 105 or 106 degrees. A throbbing headache is common, and drenching sweats are typical. The total duration of the attack averages ten to twelve hours. After malaria has persisted for up to two weeks, the disease may resolve without any medication, but recurrences may still develop as immunity is not complete. Complications of malaria include hemorrhage, anemia, and death.

In the Seventeenth Century, Jesuits in the Western Andes of South America learned of a plant bark, called chinchona, which naturally contains quinine, a hallmark in treating malaria. The amount of quinine in powdered bark varied from about one to four percent. The bark was quickly introduced into Spain, but its use in Protestant England, North America, and British possessions in the West Indies was delayed because of suspicion of Catholic treatments. Known subsequently as Jesuits' bark or Peruvian bark, it was administered following practices of the native peoples of South America. The powder commonly was prepared as a drink. Well into the Twentieth Century, quinine was the only effective drug to treat malaria.

In Jamaica, Dr. John Hunter recorded the staggering toll of tropical illnesses. The average number of deaths amounted to a fully twenty-five percent of all the British soldiers sent to the island. During his tenure spanning three years, the total number of deaths was 3,500 "without a man dying by the hands of the enemy".[3] The most common cause of death was malaria. Hunter, the military hospital superintendent, believed fevers were caused by "noxious exhalations from wet, low and marshy grounds".[4] He noted incidentally that "flies never made their appearance in any numbers, until danger, by other signs was too apparent." Despite the conscientiousness of his work, Hunter missed the causal link between malaria and mosquitos.

Benefiting immensely from hindsight, one Twentieth-Century medical author concluded, Hunter "was only one of among a number of very able men defeated not just by the time and framework within which they were operating, but by the very nature of the diseases they were studying. They were so near, and yet so far, from the discovery of mosquito transmission of yellow fever and malarias."[5] It would not be until one hundred years after the American Revolution that physicians would determine that malaria's causative micro-organism is the *Plasmodium* parasite and that it is transmitted by the Anopheles mosquito.

In his medical sleuthing, Hunter correlated the health of regiments on the island with the conditions where they were quartered. A regiment stationed near swampy ground had the worst outcomes. The island's main town of Kingston was almost as bad. He reported that twenty-eight percent of one thousand men arriving there died within the first year. Among the best stations was Stoney Hill, which was in the mountains ten miles from Kingston. There, detachments lost only "one man in twenty-six even in the height of the sickly season."[6]

Applying his observations, Hunter recommended that troops be placed in the healthy area so that England would always have "seasoned" men in the West Indies. Such men would be more valuable than twice their number sent from Europe.[7] Among his other practical recommendations, he advised sending the men on roomy transports, having them arrive in the coolest part of the year, and erecting barracks in healthy areas such as sandy, dry spots or in the mountains.[8]

An astute observer and a meticulous diarist, Hunter wrote:

> Those who are just arrived from cool and healthy climates are particularly subject to fevers ... the human frame acquires by habit a power of resisting the noxious causes.... Hence Europeans, after remaining sometime in the West Indies, are less liable to be affected by the causes of fever than on their first arrival.... The [N]egroes afford a striking example, for, though they are not entirely

> exempted from them, they suffer infinitely less than the Europeans.[9]

In these words, Hunter accurately and presciently described developing immunity to malaria.

After returning from Jamaica to London, Hunter established himself as a London practitioner and made important contributions in his own right, notably identifying lead poisoning from contaminated rum (stored in lead vessels to keep it from souring). He is also credited with the hallmark use of animal experiments in the study of infectious diseases. In recognition of his achievements, he was elected a fellow of the Royal Society and was admitted as a fellow of the College of Physicians *speciali gratia*. Hunter died in January 1809 in London.

Dr. John Rollo on St. Lucia

There were many similarities between John Hunter and John Rollo. Both were born in Scotland, educated at Edinburgh, and served in the Caribbean. Both died in 1809, Rollo eleven months after Hunter. Hunter served on St. Lucia from 1778-1779. With a force of 5,000 men, the British won over St. Lucia from the French in November 1778. British losses in the battle were small: only thirteen killed and one hundred fifty-eight wounded. But disease was so rampant that by the end of the first year, "scarcely a man remained of the original number."[10]

St. Lucia, like Jamaica was a center of the sugar trade but was smaller and had a population of just under 20,000, of whom 16,000 were enslaved persons. Like Hunter, Rollo also contributed keen observations regarding the healthier locations for troops. The healthiest was called Soufrir, which was "not exposed to the effluvia of marshes and woods"[11]. One of the worst locations was Carenage Bay, where seventeen of twenty men were sick with intermittent or relapsing fever. Eight died.

Rollo too missed the connection between mosquitos and malaria.

After two years on St. Lucia, Rollo spent another year on Barbados before returning to London. There, like Hunter, Rollo made important contributions. In 1794, he rose to Surgeon-General of the Royal Artillery. His study of diabetes led him to an important lasting recommendation. He is credited with being the first to recommend a restricted carbohydrate diet.

Drs. Hunter and Rollo served under devastating health conditions in the West Indies. Although they did not identify the mosquito as the transmitter of malaria, they both identified locations where the disease was less common. Hunter's recommendations, in and of themselves, were lifesaving.

Malaria in North America

In the late Eighteenth Century, malaria also occurred in North America, but with mercifully less devastation than in the Caribbean. Nevertheless, malaria extended even into New England in summer and fall and was especially common in the South. Officers and physicians of both armies had to deal with it in the "sickly season."

From his perspective in the Middle States, Doctor Benjamin Rush wrote that encampments next to "marshes and mill ponds let loose intermitting fevers." He also observed that winds passing "across a river before they reach [the] army ... will probably bring with them the seeds of bilious or intermitting fevers".[12] Rush made these observations keenly without knowing the underlying reason for their benefit; namely, avoidance of disease-bearing mosquitos. He, like Hunter and Rollo, also missed the connection with mosquitos.

Malaria influenced the health of the British not only in the Caribbean but also in the American South as the British tried to consolidate victories there having failed to quell the Revolution in the North. On its face, this strategy appeared to offer every opportunity as they hoped to take advantage of widespread loyalist support in the South.[13] However, changing the seat of the war created unprecedented health problems for armies on both sides fighting in North America. Fevers during the main campaigning season of summer and fall were debilitating, except in "the high country." American officers knew that as did English officers. The British commander in the South, Lord Charles Cornwallis, wrote, "The climate is so bad within one hundred miles of the coast, from June until the middle of October, that troops could not be stationed during the period without a certainty of their being rendered useless for some time for military service, if not entirely lost".[14]

The British offensive in the South began well for them with the victory at Savannah, Georgia (October 1779) and the capture of Charleston, South Carolina (May 1780). The American victor at Saratoga, General Horatio Gates, was sent South as the new commander. On route to meet the British at Camden, South Carolina, Gates's men marched through mosquito-infested marshlands and became afflicted with malaria. Weakened by disease, the Continentals were easily defeated by a stronger British army in August 1780. Gates fled and was replaced by Nathaneal Greene, Washington's favorite general.

Greene waged a war of attrition, wearing down the British and keeping his army intact. The British under General Cornwallis marched through the Carolinas and eventually into Virgina. To rest and resupply, the British encamped at Yorktown, Virgina, anticipating relief from the Royal Navy. From months of marching and fighting, Cornwallis' men were in poor health. Of his 6,618 men, a report showed 1,545 (23%) were in hospital.[15] Another source reported the number of British sick inside the Yorktown defenses as high as one-third to one-half. Fewer than 1,000 were said to be fully healthy.[16] Then disaster struck the British as a French fleet beat back the rescuing Royal Navy fleet. Cornwallis was trapped in Yorktown. A combined Franco-

American army of 16,000 marched south from New York, entered Virginia, and besieged the isolated British at Yorktown. The Crown forces under Cornwallis surrendered in October 1781. In the Allied camp, sickness was much less as about 1,400 were sick, largely from remitting fever (malaria).[17]

The surrender of Cornwallis's army at Yorktown following the surrender of Burgoyne's army at Saratoga in 1778 took the fighting will from the British. Yorktown was the last major battle of the war. Protracted peace negotiations ensued, resulting in the Treaty of Paris, signed September 1783, granting independence to the United States.

---

[1] This John Hunter is not the same person as the great Scottish surgeon, teacher, and medical author of the same name who lived 1728-1793.

[2] Wikipedia, "John Hunter (physician)", website.

[3] John Hunter, Observations on the Diseases of the Army in Jamaica, London, 1788, 70.

[4] Ibid., 39.

[5] Wilkinson.

[6] Hunter, 40.

[7] Ibid., 33.

[8] Ibid., 53.

[9] Ibid., 23.

[10] Rollo, 58.

[11] Ibid., 54.

[12] Rush, 16.

[13] Southern Loyalists supported the Crown for economic, religious and political reasons. Many Southern Loyalists were large landowners, Anglican, and conservative—all considerations opposing separation from Britain.

[14] Shanks, 278.

[15] Cantlie, 155.

[16] Shanks, 278.

[17] Duncan, 352.

CHAPTER TEN

THE ART OF MEDICAL PRACTICE IN THE EIGHTEENTH CENTURY

The art of diagnosis

The Eighteenth-Century doctor was confronted by patients with a bewildering array of fevers, rashes and eruptions, abdominal and respiratory complaints, and genital sores and discharges. At a time before stethoscopes and human thermometers were available, the physician had only his eyes and bare hands to conduct a physical examination. There were no laboratory tests to suggest or confirm the diagnosis. The doctor was simply on his own. Doctors keenly observed symptoms and findings and tried their best to categorize them into specific diagnoses.[1]

The diseases that commonly afflicted both the British and Continental armies as well as the general population were mainly infections. Although the underlying causes would not be recognized until nearly a century after the revolution, each of the diseases usually had a characteristic clinical presentation, especially as the course advanced. Through mentoring, lectures, and reading textbooks of the day, doctors passed the art of diagnosis from generation to generation.

An experienced regimental surgeon seeing a Revolutionary War soldier with a high fever, small, pale red spots, and headache would likely diagnose typhus. Alternatively, if the high fever were accompanied by pustules (small pus-filled pockets), then the diagnosis was more likely to be smallpox. If the soldier had a high fever occurring every third day, with bed-shaking chills, headache, but no rash, then the doctor likely suspected a variety of malaria. On the other hand, a Continental Army soldier with an itching rash but no fever would likely be diagnosed with simply "the itch," most often caused by scabies, but another possible diagnosis was venereal disease. Although most Eighteenth Century treatments were ineffective, making the correct diagnosis often led to life-saving interventions such as Peruvian bark for malaria and isolation early when smallpox was diagnosed.

The education of doctors

At the outbreak of the American Revolution, there were 3500 physicians in the thirteen colonies, but the odds were they never stepped foot in a medical school. Ninety percent of the physicians got their medical education through apprenticeships which were one to seven years long and were informal, unregulated training experiences under supervision by practicing doctors.

The other ten percent of doctors attended medical schools in Europe, predominantly those in London, Edinburgh, Amsterdam, Paris, Reims, Nantes, Naples, and Bologna, or in North America, but there were only two medical schools in the colonies. The first was the College of Philadelphia founded in 1765 and the forerunner of the University of Pennsylvania School of Medicine. The idea of creating the first medical school in British North America was bold and ambitious, but it worked. It was the brainchild of two visionary doctors, John Morgan, appointed Professor of Medicine, and Willam Shippen, appointed Professor of Surgery and Midwifery. They had much in common, and both were highly regarded. But they had extraordinarily different personalities, and they wound up in an intense rivalry.[2]

John Morgan (1735-1789) was brilliant and energetic but could be arrogant and egotistical. He was born in Philadelphia, and at age twenty-two years, graduated in the first class as an undergraduate from the College of Philadelphia. He then served as an apothecary resident at Pennsylvania Hospital, founded in

1751 as the first hospital in the British North American colonies. Even as an undergraduate, he studied medicine under Dr. John Redman. In the informal medical structure of the times, this was sufficient training for Morgan to serve as a surgeon during the French and Indian War (1754-1763). As customary for privileged young men of the time, he toured Europe, studying medicine in France and Italy. Morgan then traveled to Edinburgh where he entered medical school and received his medical degree in 1763. Returning to Philadelphia, Morgan was a member of the American Philosophical Society, founded in 1743 by Benjamin Franklin as the oldest learned society in the United States. His election to the society marked Morgan's standing in the scientific and intellectual community. Morgan was intent on establishing the first medical school in the British colonies.

As compared to the intense and irritable John Morgan, Doctor William Shippen (1736-1808) was affable and charming. He was also innovative. A few years before he co-founded the medical school, Shippen began the first series of lectures in America on anatomy, but his use of human bodies was unpopular with the general population. It is reported that angry mobs threw stones into his dissecting rooms. In view of his scientific contributions, Shippen also was elected to the prestigious American Philosophical Society in 1767 and became an early vice president.

The first medical class at the College of Philadelphia had only ten students. In addition to attending lectures by Drs. Morgan and Shippen, the students also received clinical instruction at Pennsylvania Hospital. According to European practice at the time, students had to purchase tickets for entering the hospital. The initial curriculum was only one year in duration and led to the degree of Bachelor of Medicine. When the curriculum was soon extended, the college provided a Doctor of Medicine.

The other medical school in the colonies at the beginning of the revolution was in New York at King's College. Founded by Dr. Samuel Bard, who invited six prominent physicians of the city to be professors in 1768, it granted its first medical degree in 1770, but most of the faculty were loyalists and left New York at the war's outbreak for Canada or England. Two others, John Jones, Professor of Surgery (see Chapter Five), and James Smith, Professor of Chemistry, supported independence and served in the Continental Army. The school closed during the city's occupation by the British beginning in 1776 and reopened in 1788, renamed Columbia Medical School.

Near the very end of the Revolutionary War, Harvard Medical School was established as the third medical school in the country in November 1782 by Doctors John Warren, brother of Doctor Joseph Warren who died at Bunker Hill, and Doctor Benjamin Waterhouse. The next medical schools to open were at Dartmouth and the University of Maryland, but not until the early Nineteenth Century.

The criteria for acceptance into American or European medical schools are not known, but as elaborated in Chapter Five, in Doctor John Jones's introduction of his textbook to students and young practitioners, he advocated for "a liberal education ... graced by the constant practice of attention tenderness, and humanity."[3]

At the time of the revolution, there was no licensing process for medical practitioners, no formal specialty training, and no specialty certification.[4]

In Eighteenth-Century North America, all physicians were white males. They wore typical Eighteenth-Century clothing, carrying out their work with bare, unwashed hands, with no knowledge that they were the spreaders of disease.[5] In the Eighteenth Century, owing to the gruesome nature of medical care—administering bleedings, emetics, and cathartics and performing ghastly operations, doctors did not have high community standing. There were great physicians who innovated and led, but many doctors were considered mere technicians. The most prestigious professions of the day were the clergy and the law.

Prior to the revolution, European physicians had published textbooks on medicine and surgery. There probably were not many copies in the colonies, but some physicians and medical faculty in North America likely used them to develop American medical practice. In 1752, Sir John Pringle, a prominent Scottish physician, published *Observations on the Diseases of the Army in Camp and Garrison*, which laid the foundation for military medicine. A subsequent text on military medicine was Donald Munro's *An Account of the Diseases which were most frequent in British Military Hospitals in Germany From January 1761 to the Return of the Troops to England in March 1763,* published in1764. Four years later, Professor of Physic and Surgery Laurence Heister wrote *A General System of Surgery*. In 1776, the renowned British physician John Hunter published *A treatise on the venereal disease*. (Note that venereal disease is singular rather than plural as syphilis and gonorrhea were then thought to be parts of the same disease.) Also in 1776, Doctor John Jones of New York published *Plain Concise Practical Remarks, on the Treatment of Wounds and Fractures*, the first medical book to be published in North America. (See Chapter Five). John Hunter's hallmark work, *A treatise on Blood, Inflammation and Gun Shot Wounds*, was published in London but not until1794.

Scientific research was in its infancy. In Great Britain, Henry Cavendish discovered hydrogen in 1766, and Joseph Priestly discovered oxygen in 1774. However, there was no organized medical research support, and medical journals in which to report scientific findings had not yet been established.[6]

The art of treatment

From a Twenty-First Century perspective, medical practices at the time of the American Revolution—bleedings, leeches, and purges—seem astonishing, confounding, or outright unthinkable. As taught to medical apprentices and medical students, the Eighteenth-Century principles of care were wrapped in the humoral theory of disease, which had prevailed from Greek and Roman times. It maintained that the body fluids or "humors" needed to be in balance for health. The four humors and their associated features were identified as: blood (linked to sanguinity, courage and optimism, hence the modern term, "sanguine"), phlegm (linked to calm and lethargy, hence the term "phlegmatic"), yellow bile (or choler, linked to short-temperedness, hence the term "choleric"), and black bile (melancholy, linked to sadness and introspectiveness). Conversely, it was believed that an imbalance of the humors caused disease. Specifically, many diseases were thought to arise from an excess of blood, considered the dominant humor. Doctors of the time believed that the body's response to infection or other severe illness (such as flushing or rapid pulse) were manifestations of excess blood. It was therefore internally consistent that, to treat disease, the balance of the humors had to be restored. Accordingly, physicians used bloodletting and leech applications to remove an excess of blood, emetics to induce vomiting, or cathartics to expel excessive bowel fluid. A low diet devoid of meat and dairy was often prescribed in addition to restore the patient's health. In the absence of a scientific basis for medical practice, these treatments persisted for centuries.

The physician had a vast array of medications in his armamentarium, but few were effective. Some were even harmful. For regimental surgeons, the Continental Army aimed to provide complete medical chests. An example from 1778 contained over twenty "Botanicals" including powdered Peruvian bark, aloe, and gum opium; five "Drugs of Animal

Origin" including cantharides (Spanish flies) and "powdered crab's eyes"; a dozen "Chemicals" including cream of tartar and calomel (mercury sulfate); three tinctures including laudanum; five ointments , including "strong mercurial ointment"; five "plasters" (adhesive bandages); a variety of surgical dressings, a set of surgical instruments, "pharmaceutical instruments" for preparing medications; and an assortment of bottles, vials, corks, and wrapping paper. Mercury as an ointment was widely used for skin ailments and orally to treat syphilis, but its toxicity was not appreciated. Ingestion of too much mercury leads to neuropsychiatric symptoms (such as headache, tremors, insomnia, and irritability), kidney failure and death. Chronic shortages of medications and supplies plagued the army for most the war.[7]

Bloodletting

Bleeding was used to treat many conditions but was mainly used for fevers due to the infections. The most common technique was venesection, that is, opening a vein. Imagine a Continental Army surgeon carrying out a bleeding on a feverish soldier with winter-time pneumonia. The surgeon opens his phlebotomy kit and takes out a large, folding lancet (also known as a fleam) with bone handles and places the sick soldier's left hand in a basin of hot water to swell the veins. He then ties a tape around the soldier's forearm. Extending the invalid's wrist, the surgeon jabs the lancet's blade into an engorged vein and extends the cut longitudinally. As the blood begins to flow, he places a pewter basin under the wrist to measure the amount. When eighteen ounces are let, the surgeon removes the tape and stops the bleeding with a dressing.

The usual volume collected for a first bleeding was twelve to forty ounces (360 to 1200 milliliters). Note that the average male's blood volume is about 160 ounces (about 5000 milliliters). The bloodletting was commonly repeated, depending on the patient's condition. Dr. John Jones was an enthusiastic supporter of bleeding. He wrote, "I scarcely need observe, that moderate evacuation, by bleeding, and gentle purging, together with a low diet, are, in these cases [wounds] absolutely necessary, ... the bleedings should be repeated at short intervals, according to the nature and urgency of the symptoms."[8]

Bleeding as a treatment could lead to dangerous complications, notably low blood pressure, shock, fainting, unconsciousness, infection, and death. Bleeding was performed repeatedly, and its use was reinforced when natural resolution of a disease occurred in conjunction with a bleeding. It was this illusion of knowledge that perpetuated the use of bleeding.[9]

Leeches

Another technique to remove blood was use of the medical leech, in Latin called *Hirudo medicinalis*. Leeches had been used for over a thousand years and were introduced into European practice in the Middle Ages. Leeches, which are related biologically to earthworms, are found in nature, living in water and feeding on decaying plants. They attach to the human skin by a bite, but it is not painful because leech saliva contains a local anesthetic. Through its proboscis, the leech absorbs human blood.

In the Continental Army, leeches were not listed in the contents of regimental medical chests[10] making it unlikely that regimental surgeons had access to them in the field. Leeches would probably have been available in the general hospital for use at the doctors' discretion. Picture then a senior physician caring for an infantry lieutenant who was suffering from an infected gunshot wound of his leg. If the lieutenant has not improved with one or more venesections, then leeches are in order. The senior physician selects from his medical case a sterling thumb forceps, reaches into a ceramic jar, and brings out the first brown leech. It is about three inches long and a half-inch wide. Its round head is about a quarter inch in diameter. The doctor applies the first leeches to the lieutenant's left posterior chest wall so that the officer could not see them. Then he places four more. The next morning the leeches are swollen with blood, each one now a dark red-purple color and ten times its original size. Each leech removes about ten milliliters (one-third of an ounce) of blood. There is redness around the attachment sites. Because the leeches are full, the doctor plucks them off with his thumb forceps. At the attachment sites, there are small oozing ulcers to which the doctor applies lint and a cloth bandage.[11]

Purgatives and Emetics

Laxatives, also called purgatives or cathartics, and emetics also were commonly used to restore the balance to body humors. Physicians had many choices of laxative medications effective in evacuating the bowels and inducing diarrhea.[12] Among these were the biologicals (jalap root, rhubarb, snakeroot ["seneka"] and castor oil) and the chemicals (Glauber's salt, Plummer's pills, and Epsom salts). Glauber was a Seventeenth Century physician and chemist, who prepared a salt of sodium sulfate hydrate. Plummer's pills were named for an Eighteenth-Century Scottish physician, who prepared a mixture of calomel (a mercury compound), antimony sulfide, and guaiacum (from a flowering evergreen tree). Plummer's pills were originally used to treat syphilis but also worked as a purge. Epsom salts, made up of magnesium sulfate, are named after the famed English baths. The most common medications to induce vomiting were ipecac from a South American plant and tartar emetic. Serious complications could accompany these therapies. Especially in febrile patients, they could lead to severe dehydration and shock. In addition, some of the chemicals, especially ones containing mercury, are very toxic, as discussed above.[13]

Medications

From the long list of medications used, here is a description of the most common ones. A few of those effective drugs are still used today in some form.

The bark

As described in Chapter Nine, chinchona bark, known then as Jesuits' bark or Peruvian bark, naturally contains quinine, a hallmark in treating malaria. During the revolution, both armies were using Peruvian bark not only for malaria but often for other fevers as well. It was used by the ton resulting in a quadrupling of its price. The major American source of the bark had been importation from Britain. Once that source was eliminated with the start of the war, Americans faced a critical shortage of this life-saving natural medication. Surprisingly, the most important source in the early years of the war was American privateers who captured drug cargoes in British prize ships. Privateers from Massachusetts captured over 1000 cargo ships. Privateers were individuals authorized by a government to attack foreign ships. In 1777, one of these prize ships carried four tons of chinchona bark.[14] American agents in Europe also would have been able to purchase the bark from allied countries. Yet these were stopgap measures barely meeting the army's needs. Not until after the alliance with France in February 1778 was the medical supply shortage finally resolved. As part of a broad strategy to undermine British power, the French directly supplied and transported medical supplies to the Continental Army and also provided financial aid to obtain medicines from other sources.

Well into the Twentieth Century, quinine was the only effective anti-malaria drug. In the Twenty-First Century, many species of the malaria parasite have developed resistance to quinine, but an array of other drugs is available for prevention and treatment of malaria.

Laudanum and gum opium

First created in the Sixteenth Century, laudanum contains opium powder dissolved in alcohol. It comes from the poppy plant and has a very bitter taste. This was the first available effective pain killer and was used for battlefield wounds, during surgery, and for a variety of diseases. Because it slowed intestinal motion, laudanum was also used to treat diarrhea from dysentery. Laudanum became widely used in the colonies at the time of the revolution but was soon recognized as being highly addictive. Its common side effects are itching, mood changes, and contracted eye pupils ("pinpoint pupils"). When taken in large doses, it may cause respiratory suppression and death.[15] Gum opium was another narcotic preparation used as an alternative to laudanum. It is a brownish sticky fluid that oozes from unripe seedpods of the opium poppy.

Belladonna

Belladonna comes from the plant, the Deadly Nightshade (in Latin, *Atropa belladonna*). The name belladonna means "beautiful lady" in Italian, based upon the plant's use as a cosmetic in ancient times. In the Eighteenth Century, belladonna was used to treat abdominal cramps and diarrhea. It was commonly administered as a powder often in a soothing combination such as with honey and licorice. However, even in small doses, it had numerous, common side effects such as drowsiness, dry mouth, impaired vision, constipation, muscle spasms, and overheating. Further, as the name Deadly Nightshade indicates, it is highly toxic and poisonous. Serious side effects are fever, rapid heart rate, hallucinations, and seizures. The alternative medication to treat the flux was opium, but this could cause marked drowsiness and marked sedation.[16]

Wine

Wine was used widely for its many properties, as a sedative for an anxious or pre-operative soldier and even as a substitute for treating malaria when there was a shortage of the bark.

Poultices, ointments, and salves

Skin afflictions consisting of rashes, ulcers, blisters, infected cuts or insect bites, and pustules were everyday problems for the common soldier. In an era before good hygiene and precise diagnostics, Revolutionary War doctors applied a variety of soothing treatments. A bread and milk poultice (a moist application of a comforting material) was commonly used since it was easy to prepare and made of available components. Crumbled bread was stirred into boiling milk, cooled, and spread on a cloth. It was often mixed with lard and smeared on the affected parts. Doctors used a variety of ointments. Ingredients which may have brought effective relief in these unguents were "calamine stone" (which contains a healing zinc compound and is the basis of modern calamine lotion), aloe, and camphor.

Other medicinals

With the best of intentions, Eighteenth Century physicians searched for still other medications to relieve suffering, often turning to herbs, plants, and chemicals, found either locally or imported. In addition to those described above, doctors applied "bitter apple" (colocynth) and "Indian pokeweed" (Hellebore) as purgatives, wintergreen as a urinary irritant, and tragacanth gum as an adhesive. Cantharides, prepared from dried insects notably Spanish flies, were used as a counterirritant in blistering plasters. This medication had formerly been used as an aphrodisiac. A preparation exotically called "powdered crab's eyes" is from crayfish stomachs and is a source of calcium. It was used to treat ulcers and fevers.

Medicine Leaps into the Scientific Era

With the benefit of hindsight, it is easy to be critical of the entire system of medical education and practice of the Eighteenth-Century Western world. It is tempting to disparage physicians for not rising above their time and place and for continuing to ply their craft with harmful bleedings, leeches, cathartics, and emetics. Yet, as described in the extensive footnotes, medical science and practice began its giant leap into a scientific era about fifty to seventy years after the American Revolution. Those advances based upon anatomy, chemistry, epidemiology, and microbiology led to vast progress in diagnosis and treatment, but they came too late for the men and women who fought for American independence.

---

[1] Today, the doctor elicits specific complaints and findings and must decide on a most likely diagnosis and other diagnostic possibilities as well. In modern medicine, the list of possible causes is called the differential diagnosis. Medical practice remains hard because of the uncertainty in the decision-making. As Osler noted over a century ago, "Medicine is a science of uncertainty and an art of probability" (Osler, 1903, Cited in Longo et al, *Harrison's Principles of Internal Medicine*, Chapter 4: Decision-Making in Clinical Medicine, 2022). An authoritative, current textbook of medicine recognizes these ongoing challenges. Clinical diagnosis is a quest, putting together all the symptoms, findings and tests, and reassessing when the fit doesn't seem to work out. Diagnosis in the practice of medicine remains a "craft" or an art as well as a science (Longo). Today's doctors are supported in their hunt for a diagnosis by sophisticated imaging tests such as magnetic resonance imaging (MRIs) and computed tomography (CTs) and by thousands of laboratory tests from complete blood counts (CBCs) to reference assays for rare diseases. To aid in diagnosis, doctors now have clinical "decision support" tools using the internet and very recently artificial intelligence. Coming up with the right diagnosis is essential in modern medicine when we have effective treatments for most diseases and excellent infection control measures for contagious illnesses.

[2] Reiss, 55-67.

Notes, continued

---

[3] Jones, 5.

[4] Medical education changed dramatically when the scientific basis of practice was established and standards for medical school accreditation and medical licensing were accepted in the late Nineteenth and early Twentieth Century. In the modern era, entry into medical school requires at least a bachelor's degree and is extremely competitive. The overall acceptance rate for American medical schools is 44.5% with the rate varying widely among schools. Top tier schools have acceptance rates below 10%. The medical school curriculum lasts four years including both basic medical science courses (such as anatomy, physiology, biochemistry, and pharmacology) and clinical rotations through the specialties (such as internal medicine, surgery, pediatrics, obstetrics and gynecology, and family medicine). At graduation from medical school, the new doctor receives the MD degree. Nearly all MDs continue their education by taking residency programs in their chosen field. Officially called graduate medical education programs, residencies generally require three to seven years of rigorous training. Following residency, a physician takes an examination, called specialty boards, to qualify for specialty certification. Some physicians take even further training, called fellowships to become "subspecialists." In internal medicine, examples would include cardiology or infectious diseases. In my specialty of obstetrics and gynecology, the subspecialties include gynecologic cancer, reproductive endocrinology and infertility, and high-risk obstetrics (called Maternal Fetal Medicine). Today, medical licensing requires passing a state or national examination. Hospital privileges, meaning the ability to admit patients and perform procedures, are granted by individual hospitals or hospital systems. Board certification is commonly required to be granted hospital privileges. Thus, today's physicians go through an educational and vetting process that takes up to a decade or more after entering medical school. High standards are enforced to maintain quality of care.

[5] The first woman to graduate from an American medical school was Elizabeth Blackwell, who graduated from Geneva Medical College (in New York State) in 1849. The first Black American to get a medical degree was James McCune Smith, and he had to go to Scotland for his degree from the University of Glasgow in 1837.There were no white coats, no scrub suits, no operating gowns, no masks, and no gloves. The concept of sterilization would come with the contributions of Joseph Lister in Scotland in the 1860s.

[6] Today, medical research is a giant entity with an annual budget in the United States of $161 billion dollars. Funding comes from the federal government mainly through the National Institutes of Health (founded in1887) with its budget of $48 billion and from industry and private foundations. Most research is reported in medical journals which began in 1797. The oldest

Notes, continued

general medical journals still published today are *The New England Journal of Medicine*, established in 1812, and *The Lancet*, in 1823. Today, it is estimated that, world-wide, there are 15,000 influential medical journals publishing nearly a million articles annually.

[7] Griffenhagen.

[8] Jones, 24-26.

[9] Medical reports on the ineffectiveness and danger of bleeding appeared in about 1830, but the practice continued even into the later part of the Nineteenth Century. In modern practice, bleeding is reserved for rare conditions such as polycythemia vera, in which there is a dangerously high blood count, and hemochromatosis, in which there is an excess of iron in the body.

[10] Griffenhagen.

[11] Leech saliva contains numerous substances including anticoagulants, anti-inflammatories, and anesthetics. Leech therapy was abandoned in the Nineteenth Century but has been re-introduced into practice in the last few decades—but for entirely different reasons. Taking advantage of the anticoagulants and other substances in leech saliva, doctors may currently use leeches to remove blood clots from wounds or pus from an abscess.

[12] Griffenhagen.

[13] In modern practice, laxatives are used for constipation and bowel preparation before diagnostic or surgical procedures. Emetics may be used after accidental ingestion of poisons.

[14] Parascondola.

[15] In recent years, other opium derivatives were excessively used for pain syndromes leading to a sharp rise in death rates from overdosing. In response, practice changes included provider and patient education, prescription of smaller numbers of opiate pills, and use of alternative non-opiate medication. As a result, overdose deaths in the United States fell sharply. Between 2023 and 2024, the Centers for Disease Control reported that deaths due to fentanyl (a synthetic opioid) dropped 36% from 76,000 to 48,000, and cocaine deaths fell 28% from 31,000 to 22,000.

[16] Belladonna may be used in modern medicine to treat spasm of the ureter (the tubular structure leading from kidney to bladder). Safer medications are available to treat diarrhea.

CHAPTER ELEVEN

AFFLICTIONS OF GENERALS, ADMIRALS, STATESMEN, AND THE KING: THE LIMITATION OF MEDICAL PRACTICE AND ITS CONSEQUENCES

With the background on the diagnosis and treatment in the Eighteenth Century (Chapter Ten), we now turn to case studies to see how these limitations of medical practice played out even among the powerful. Because of privileged living conditions, officers and statesmen were usually spared the ravages of some infections such as typhus, but the upper classes were subject to gout (from their diet rich in red meat and alcohol), chronic abdominal disorders, and mental conditions. In some case studies, the diagnosis was correct, but treatment was either wrong (by modern standards) or limited. In other cases, the diagnosis eluded the best medical minds of the times, and treatment was ineffective. Because severe illness incapacitated governmental officials and military officers at critical times, history raises several intriguing questions about what outcomes in the war's course might have changed if the notables had been in good health. For many of the figures sketched below, there are pertinent *what if?* questions.

The Americans

Benjamin Franklin (1706-1790)

Despite debilitating illness, Benjamin Franklin overwhelmingly managed through his personal discipline to fulfill his civic obligations. He has been called "the greatest diplomat that America ever had",[1] but he suffered from gout and bladder stones so severely that it periodically impaired his ability to attend to public duties. Because of its characteristic findings, the diagnosis of gout was often made accurately in the Eighteenth Century.[2]

Born in Boston in 1706, he was an accomplished publisher and printer, activist, military organizer, philosopher, and scientist. Franklin was an early advocate for smallpox inoculation, especially following the death of his six-year-old son Francis from natural smallpox in 1736.[3] He raised funds to establish Pennsylvania Hospital, in Philadelphia, and served on its board. As a scientist, Franklin charted the Gulf Stream, experimented with electricity, and invented bifocal glasses. On top of these diverse achievements, Franklin left his lasting mark on American history through his extraordinary skills as a diplomat in Europe. For fifteen years, he served as the colonial agent for Pennsylvania in London prior to the revolution, and after the war broke out, he served as the country's senior diplomat in Europe. There, he played the lead in negotiating the critical Franco-American alliance in 1778. In the next three years until the culminating victory at Yorktown, Franklin maintained the alliance, successfully getting French financial aid, armaments, and army and naval support. His achievements are even more impressive in view of his advanced age and "crippling bouts" of gout, severe pain from a bladder stone, and a troublesome skin condition, most likely psoriasis.

Franklin's gout had its onset when he was in his forties. Attacks of his hands, feet, and knees made him bedridden on occasion. While in Paris, gout so limited his mobility that he needed a wheelchair at times. After an especially painful attack on October 22, 1780, he wrote a satirical work, entitled "Dialogue Between Franklin and the Gout," in which he identified eating and drinking too freely as the cause.[4] The painful bladder stones almost certainly were a consequence of his gout. Surgeons at the time "cut for stone" (that is, operated to remove bladder stones), but Franklin never had the procedure. First, his stone may have been too large for removal, and second there was a high risk of infection and death from the procedure, especially at his age. Franklin managed his pain as best as he could with diet (low in red meat and in alcohol) and in his last years with opium.

Although, at times, the combination of the great sage's afflictions affected his ability to attend a formal function or event, the resilient and energetic Franklin persevered. He never let his gout prevent him from achieving his tasks. Historian Edward Larson recognizes Franklin, along with Washington, as one of the two the most important Founding Fathers.[5]

He returned to America after the war and in 1787 was effective in crafting a strong central government at the Constitutional Convention in Philadelphia. Three years later, the American genius was bedridden and developed pneumonia, which claimed his life on April 17,1790 at age eighty-four years.

General Nathaneal Greene (1742-1786)

In contrast to Benjamin Franklin, General Nathaneal Greene's medical conditions arguably raise legitimate "what if" questions. Acclaimed as one of Washington's best generals, Nathaneal Greene suffered from two recurring medical conditions. One bout of illness incapacitated him just before a critical battle in 1776 and possibly altered the course of the war. Greene was a Rhode Islander from a Quaker family. In 1773, shortly after being expelled by the Quakers, reportedly for visiting a tavern, he began his military career by joining a militia unit.[6] In May 1775, the Rhode Island assembly voted to raise a brigade and appointed Nathaneal Greene as brigadier general, based not only upon family connections but also his looming military potential. By age thirty-four years, he was appointed as the youngest brigadier general in the Continental Army and quickly became Washington's favorite. Just under six feet tall, with broad shoulders and a stout chest, he was decisive, disciplined, and devoted to Washington.[7] From a childhood injury, he had a pronounced limp, but it did not interfere with his effectiveness or advancement.

In January 1776, while in the American army surrounding Boston, Greene developed his first episode of fever, jaundice, and malaise. In early February, he wrote, "I am as yellow as saffron, my appetite all gone and my flesh too. I am so weak that I can scarcely walk across the room".[8] His wife Caty, heavy with child, came from Rhode Island to nurse him back to health.

He recovered but eight months later, during the actions around New York, Greene was incapacitated by another similar bout. Greene, just promoted to Major General and in command of the army's defenses on Long Island (Brooklyn), became ill on August 15th, as the British were preparing to attack the American position.[9] Greene, bed-ridden with a raging fever, nausea, vomiting, and abdominal pains, was removed to a home on Manhattan to recuperate.

With the trustworthy Greene out of action, command in Brooklyn fell to newly promoted Major General John Sullivan, but Washington found him wanting and appointed fifty-eight-year-old Major General Israel Putnam to command. In just five days, the front had three American commanders. In part because of poor intelligence about the British plan of attack, the Americans were routed at Brooklyn with great losses of killed, wounded and captured. In his sickbed in Manhattan, Greene, still terribly weak, wept at the news. (I found no record of what his doctors thought he had nor how they treated him.)

What was going on with Greene during these episodes in 1776? Recurrent bouts of weakness, fever, abdominal pain, either with or without jaundice, occurring in an otherwise young, healthy officer suggest several diagnostic possibilities. Leading causes include acute cholecystitis (inflammation of the gall bladder due to stones), hepatitis, pancreatitis (inflammation of the pancreas gland), and less likely malaria.

It is tempting to ask *what if?* Greene had remained in command. Would the disaster on Long Island have been averted? Would the entire campaign in New York have turned out differently? In the end of August, Greene wrote, "I have not the vanity to think the event would have been otherwise had I been there, yet I could have given the commanding general a good deal of necessary information".[10] Another senior American officer wrote, "We had one chance and only one for the defense of New York ... had General Greene been fit for duty I flatter myself matters would have worn a very different appearance at present".[11] Greene almost certainly would have foreseen and planned for the flanking attack that resulted in the American defeat with 200 killed and wounded and nearly 1,000 patriot soldiers captured and sent to British prison ships where many of them would die of disease. What saved the rest of the American army was the almost miraculous escape under cover of a sudden fog that descended over the East River and allowed several thousand troops to escape to temporary safety in Manhattan.

Greene also had recurring asthma which he wrote about in several letters. Just prior to the Battle of the Brandywine (September 11, 1777), he wrote to his wife that sleeping in a dusty bed gave him asthma and made it difficult to sleep, but he was able to fight during the long battle the next day on a field shrouded in heavy smoke from tens of thousands of muskets plus artillery.

The next year, in August 1778, while in Rhode Island, he wrote to her that he had been "a little troubled by the asthma but have gotten over it".[12] The next day, his asthma worsened. In a report of the Battle of Rhode Island on August 29, 1778, he added, "I am very much unwell, have had no sleep for three Nights & Days; being severely afflicted with the Asthma."

Washington appointed Greene as Southern Commander after the British victory at Camden (August 1780), but Greene was so ill that he requested additional time before taking command "having had a considerable fever upon me for several days." While in command in the South, Greene, like Franklin, fought through his illness and was an effective commander.

After the war, Greene settled in Georgia and died of sunstroke in June 1786 after walking in a neighbor's field. He was just forty-three years old.

General Charles Lee (1732-1782)

When most of us hear of "General Lee," our thoughts go to the Virginian general of the Civil War, but General Charles Lee could not have been more different from Robert E. Lee. Charles Lee was English by birth, served as an officer in the British Army, was a soldier of fortune in Europe, and in the early 1770s embraced American independence. He even became second in command to Washington. Yet Charles Lee remains in the shadows of history. Contemporaries and historians described him as "insane, or at least subject to madness".[13] Lee's entire career was marked by repeated physical illnesses and, to be generous, an unusual personality, especially for an Eighteenth-Century officer. Physically, he was rail thin with an "ugly face".[14] Because of his large nose, fellow officers called him "Naso" behind his back. He loved to be with his dogs more often than with people.[15] Although he had relationships with several women, they were "unblessed by state and church, except in the case of his Iroquois wife".[16] Based upon his outbursts, the Native Americans nicknamed him "boiling water."

His military career began as a British officer in North America and Europe in the early 1750s-1760s and then continued in Poland where he was commissioned as a major general in the Polish Army. While in Europe, he developed his first crippling bouts of rheumatism or gout in 1766 and became "desperately ill—delirious for eight days and given up for lost for three weeks".[17] While in France, he suffered from "distemper of the brain." Yet he recovered fully from these illnesses and, by late 1773, made his way to North America. Armed with an introductory letter from Benjamin Franklin, he met with Thomas Jefferson and was hosted by the Washingtons. When the Revolutionary War broke out, Congress, impressed with his record, appointed him major general, second in command to Washington. However, Lee thought more highly of his own military skills than of Washington's, and on occasion intentionally disobeyed Washington's orders.

In early 1776, Lee was put in charge of the defenses of New York. Recurring gout or rheumatism struck again. He was "unable to walk, suffered great pain, ran a fever, and could not sleep nor eat for eight days".[18] After he recovered, Lee was sent to Charleston to defend against the British sea-borne invasion. There, he quarreled with Carolina militia officers who resented his arrogance.[19]Upon returning to New York, he argued with another senior officer about the defenses along the Hudson River.

After the loss of Fort Washington in November 1776, support for General Washington reached a low ebb. Lee put the blame for this disaster directly on Washington in a "bitterly, recklessly, despairingly" written letter to his friend General Horatio Gates.[20] Lee pictured himself accepting supreme command of the Continental Army. However, Washington rode out the storm, and Lee's career began to plummet. What if Washington had had Lee's command experience rather than having to learn from so many mistakes? Would the series of early American losses have been averted? Or, what if Lee had not had the personality disorder that put him in conflict with Washington and prevented a healthy collaboration between the two commanders?

In December 1776, Lee was captured by the British and, as a prisoner of war, proposed to end the war with "a quick and almost bloodless British victory with generous terms for the

Americans".[21] One modern historian defended Lee's proposal as "not intrinsically immoral; nor was it impractical." However, if Lee's plan had become known to the Americans, "it is not unlikely that he would have been found guilty of treachery and sentenced to death".[22] As it turned out, Lee was exchanged in 1778 and took command of an American wing at the Battle of Monmouth, New Jersey in June 1778. There, he ordered an untimely retreat, infuriating Washington. At a subsequent court martial, Lee was found guilty and suspended from command in the army.

In September 1782, he became so ill from fever and lung disease that he drew up his final will. On October 2nd, "in a final fit of delirium ... his racked body and troubled spirit gave up the fight".[23]

What was Lee's psychiatric diagnosis? He was learned (able to read Greek), worldly, tireless, ambitious, and at times charming. On the dark side, he was a difficult person: quarrelsome, arrogant, resentful, slovenly, profane, promiscuous, impulsive, and melancholy. Looking back 250 years, a modern psychiatrist would have a difficult time making a firm diagnosis, but with the wide mood swings of his life, Charles Lee might well have had bipolar disease, previously called manic depressive disorder.

General Philip Schuyler (1733-1804)

Philip Schuyler was a member of New York's Dutch American aristocracy who had gained wealth from land ownership.[24] In 1755, Schuyler married Catherine van Rensselaer, of another upper-crust, landowning family. Together they had fifteen children, but only eight survived into their adult years. Schuyler had another famous family connection. He was Alexander Hamilton's father-in-law and held Hamilton as closely as family and in high regard.

In June 1775, General Washington put Schuyler in command of the New York Department of the Continental Army. In that post, Schuyler planned the two-armed invasion of Canada. (See Chapter One.) As major general, he led the American forces marching northward through New York to attack Montreal, but he developed such severe "rheumatic gout" that he had to give up command. He wrote to Philadelphia, "I am so low as not to be able to hold a pen".[25] General Richard Montgomery replaced him, led the capture of Montreal, but was mortally wounded in December 1775 during the disastrous American attack on Quebec. Had Schuyler been healthy and retained command, his judicious nature might have avoided the forlorn attack on Quebec and averted the heavy losses of American troops there. Schuyler remained in Upstate New York and in spring 1776 met the Americans retreating from Canada. He led them southward on the retreat. Because he gave up Fort Ticonderoga to the pursuing British, he was subject to court martial but was acquitted.

In 1777, Schuyler was healthy and with American General Horatio Gates planned the campaign against the British invasion from Canada, under General Burgoyne. Elitist and aristocratic, Schuyler was unpopular with the New England soldiers, and he feuded with Gates. Schuyler complained to Congress, which supported him. Schuyler then rallied the troops from Upstate New York and was "forced to work closely" with Gates.[26] The two American generals overcame their feuding and oversaw the American victory at Saratoga. In the Eighteenth Century, high-ranking officers of both sides considered each other with collegiality. After Burgoyne's surrender in October 1777, Schuyler hosted him as a prisoner of war at Schuyler's mansion in Albany. For the next two years, Schuyler continued to quarrel with Congress surrounding his court martial and finally resigned in 1779.

Afterwards, Schuyler had a prominent personal and political career. He remained close with the Washingtons, who were the godparents to the Schuyler's youngest daughter.[27] Schuyler was appointed to the New York State Board of Regents in 1784. A strong Federalist, he supported the constitution's ratification and became New York's first senator in 1789. Poor health marked his second term in the United States Senate, and he died in November 1804.

The British

King George III (1738-1820)

The king's mental symptoms were so well known that they became the subject of a 1994 British film, *The* Madness *of King George III*, a comedy drama, but in fairness we need to provide the full story.

George III became king in 1760 at age twenty-two years. Although he had periods of mental aberration, the king had an inquisitive mind. He was fascinated by maps and the solar system[28] and had a huge collection of scientific instruments. During his sixty-year reign, he was a patron of the serious arts and "defied the vicious prejudices of the day against homosexuality and bisexuality".[29] He had fifteen children.

The king's symptoms began five years after his inauguration with the first attack lasting from January to July 1765. During this period, parliament debated having the colonists pay for the costs of the French and Indian War. On March 22, 1765, parliament passed the Stamp Act, which was the beginning of the government's series of repressive laws. The hard line taken by George III and his ministers led to open rebellion a decade later. The king's constellation of physical and mental symptoms may have affected his policy-making in the lead up to the revolution. Intermittent attacks occurred after the war up until his death in 1820. Each of the attacks was complex, according to one modern analysis,[30] beginning with cold, cough, and malaise, followed in the first attack by "stitches in the breast" and in others by crampy abdominal pain and constipation, rapid heart rate, hoarseness, weakness and stiffness. Some episodes included tremor, foaming at the mouth, speechlessness, and incontinence. Mental symptoms were prominent: agitation, non-stop and vehement talking, uninhibited behavior, nighttime confusion, insomnia, delusions, hallucinations, and extraordinary excitement, including violence and abusiveness.[31,32] As concerning as these symptoms were, they abated suddenly and at one time did not recur for twelve years.

Worried and perplexed contemporary royal physicians labelled His Royal Highness as having "delirium" or simply "insanity". The king was treated with restraints but rarely with the sedating drug laudanum.[33] He was also subject to medical regimens of the day: emetics, bleedings, purges, and leeches. At the end, George was blind, deaf, and impaired.

George III's illness alarmed members of Parliament and government ministers. Well after his death in1820, his illness fascinated Nineteenth and Twentieth Century physicians who generated the various posthumous diagnosis of "acute mania," manic-depressive psychosis (today called bipolar disease), or "neurotic personality".[34] In 1966, two British psychiatrists reviewed new records, weighed George's physical symptoms and findings more heavily, and proposed an altogether novel diagnosis: acute intermittent porphyria.[35] This is a rare, hereditary disorder of heme (a component of hemoglobin) metabolism. The disease leads to a buildup of toxic compounds and causes a wide array of physical and neurologic symptoms, including those shown by the king. This diagnosis was widely accepted for nearly fifty years until effectively challenged in 2010 by two English scholars.[36] Blasting the 1966 work, point-by-point, the more recent analysis argues that "the porphyria diagnosis was based on weak foundations, bolstered by indiscriminate aggregation of symptoms and suppression of contrary indicators. It appears very unlikely that the King was suffering from porphyria and therefore the causes of his 'madness' remain "an unsolved mystery".[37]

William Pitt the Elder (1708-1778)

For the great British statesman, William Pitt the Elder (1708-1778), also known as the First Earl of Chatham, gout's onset occurred when he was a child.[38,39] He served as Prime Minister and is credited with successfully managing the Seven Years' War (The French and Indian War) for England. Yet, the gouty attacks were so severe during his career that they limited his impact. Pitt also suffered from mental health problems and had a "nervous breakdown" while Prime Minister.[40] As a member of the opposition in 1765, he opposed the Stamp Act but missed critical debates in 1765 due to illness. Historians have asked *what if?* Pitt had been healthy and present for the Parliamentary debate. Would Pitt's brilliance have defeated passage of the Stamp Act which was the first Parliamentary move leading to the American Revolution? Would Parliament have adopted an accommodating stance for its American colonies? Could the revolution have been avoided? Ten years later, when the war broke out, Pitt was a strong supporter of the Americans' position. His end came dramatically in May 1778. In one account of his last moments, he died in the arms of his son, William Pitt the Younger, who was reading to him from Homer. In the other version, he collapsed on the floor of Parliament during a speech. He was buried in Westminster Abbey with full British pomp.

Admiral George Rodney (1718-1792)

The story of George Bridges Rodney's afflictions gives us an even more enticing *what if?* scenario. Born into an upper-crust English family, Rodney joined the navy at just fifteen years of age. Taking advantage of family influence and his own prowess, he rose rapidly and became an admiral by age forty-one.[41] After his successful exploits against the French in the Caribbean in the 1760s, he was made a baronet and then became a member of Parliament, but all was not going well for Rodney. "Profligate gambling, spending, and womanizing ... lead to severe indebtedness," and his arrogance and contemptuousness made him unpopular in the upper ranks of the Royal Navy. What's more, from his time in the tropics he had been troubled with malaria, and like many peers he developed severe episodes of gout.

In 1779, fearful of French and Spanish involvement in the Americas, the Admiralty placed Rodney, now sixty-one-years-old and out of naval action for sixteen years, in command of the Barbados station. There, additional gout attacks debilitated him, but he performed well. In 1781, a new medical problem beset him: painful and difficult urination, attributed by his doctor to a stricture of the urethra (the passage leading from the bladder through the penis). Also suffering from the gout, Rodney wrote to Lord Sandwich, First Lord of the Admiralty, in England requesting to return to England for medical care. Permission arrived in August 1781, and the victorious, competent Admiral Rodney immediately left for England. He was replaced by Admiral Thomas Graves just as the French fleet under Admiral de Grasse was sailing from the Caribbean toward its historic rendezvous in Chesapeake Bay just off Yorktown, Virginia. Graves sailed to challenge the French and to relieve the isolated British Army in Yorktown under General Cornwallis. But Graves was no Rodney. He was described as an "elderly, incompetent political appointee," with limited skills in naval tactics.[42]The French fleet got the favorable position in the bay, and Graves delayed his attack. In the ensuing battle on September 5, 1781, the British sustained heavy damage, but lost no ships, before nightfall ended the action. Graves chose not to renew the battle the next day, but sailed back to New York, leaving the trapped Cornwallis and his army of 7,000 on their own. Graves planned to organize a larger relief force in New York, but by the time they sailed, the successful Franco-American siege had already led to Cornwallis's surrender at Yorktown on October 19th.

The tempting question is: *What if* Rodney had been healthy and in command? Would he have done better? Would he have been able to drive off the French and either reinforce or evacuate Cornwallis, avoiding the war ending surrender at Yorktown? The British were somewhat outgunned, with nineteen ships of the line and 1410 cannon compared with twenty-four French ships of the line with 1542 cannon. Nevertheless, a bolder Royal Navy admiral like Rodney, might have shown superior tactics and saved the day—and the war for the king. This is not purely fanciful thinking. Rodney faced de Grasse the next year in the Caribbean and beat him (as described below).

As for Rodney, he arrived in England in late September, took care of financial matters, and sought care from an eminent surgeon, Sir Caesar Hawkins, who dilated Rodney's urethra. The procedure, performed without anesthesia, must have been dreadfully painful. At the time, most urethral strictures were thought to be consequences of venereal disease, and we know today that gonorrhea causes such strictures. Rodney was reported to be a womanizer. It is presumed that Rodney's surgery was successful because three weeks later the Admiralty appointed him in command of the Atlantic fleet. He set sail in January 1782 and fought de Grasse off the coast of Dominica in Mid-April. Using new tactics that Lord Horatio Nelson used later at Trafalgar, Rodney won "a most complete Victory".[43]

Admiral Richard Howe (1726-1799)

Admiral Lord Richard Howe, the older brother of General William Howe and commander of the British Fleet in America during the revolution, was afflicted by gout for over thirty years. The painful bouts do not appear to have limited his activity during the revolution, but in his last years he needed crutches even to walk at home. His death was due to complications of gout.

Treatment Limitations and *What Ifs*

In the brief medical histories presented here, we have examples of illness taking from command positions American General Greene, American General Schuyler, and British

Admiral Rodney. As evidenced by the limited success in the treatment of even the notables and the wealthy of the Revolutionary War, the best medical training often failed to help patients. These outcomes raise legitimate *what if?* questions. Would the outcome of battles in Canada, Long Island or Yorktown have been different if these commanders had been healthy? And then we saw how statesmen like the great William Pitt of England and the incomparable Benjamin Franklin of America were not always able to share their voices at certain discussions and functions to which they otherwise would have contributed their wisdom. The history of the American Revolution is marked by the convergence of medicine and war, and it teases us to engage with all the medical *what ifs?*

---

[1] Larson, 145-146, quote attributed to historian Gordon Wood.

[2] With its hallmark findings of exquisitely painful inflammation of usually one (but sometimes more) joint, notably of the great toe, gout has been recognized since ancient times. Its manifestations include not only painful arthritis, but also urinary tract stones. Because it has been long associated with rich foods and excessive alcohol, gout has been referred to as "the disease of kings." Three thousand years ago, Hippocrates accurately described it. In 1697, using his newly invented microscope, van Leuwenhoek saw crystals in gouty deposits of the affected joints. By the late Eighteenth Century, these crystals were identified as uric acid. Treatment at the time of the revolution included poultices, bloodletting, purgatives, opioids, and many herbal medications. Colchicine, prepared from the autumn crocus flower, had been used for centuries to treat gout, but it was abandoned in the Eighteenth Century because of adverse gastrointestinal side-effects when used in high doses. In the early Nineteenth Century, colchicine was reintroduced and has remained a mainstay in modern times. Today, gout is recognized as the result of abnormal metabolism of uric acid, and it is treated with drugs to decrease inflammation (colchicine, steroids, or nonsteroidals such as ibuprofen) or to limit episodes by decreasing uric acid levels (allopurinol). Recommended lifestyle changes include limiting red meat and alcohol and keeping well hydrated.

[3] Gensel, 536-537.

[4] Mikhail and Siva.

[5] Larson, 145-146.

[6] Physical challenges of ... Greene, website.

Notes, continued

---

[7] Atkinson, I, 450.

[8] Physical challenges of ... Greene, website.

[9] Atkinson, I, 358.

[10] Physical challenges of ... Greene, website.

[11] Physical challenges of ... Greene, website.

[12] Physical challenges of ... Greene, website.

[13] Alden, 304-305.

[14] Alden, 304-305.

[15] Alden, 77-78.

[16] Alden, 304-305.

[17] Alden, 27-28, 37, 45.

[18] Alden, 97-98.

[19] Alden, 123-4, 134, 142, 147.

[20] Ibid.

[21] Alden, 178, 238, 298.

[22] Ibid.

[23] Ibid.

[24] C. D. McE. Ingraham, "Philip John Schuyler", *The Digital Encyclopedia of George Washington*, MountVernon.org website.

[25] Atkinson, I, 147.

[26] Ingraham, "Philip John Schuyler", MountVernon.org website.

[27] Ibid.

[28] Roberts, 112.

[29] Roberts, 227.

[30] MacAlpine.

[31] MacAlpine.

[32] Roberts, 521-23.

[33] Roberts, 521-23.

[34] MacAlpine.

[35] Ibid.

[36] Peters and Wilkinson.

[37] Ibid.

[38] Dunea.

[39] Atkinson, I, 72, 176-77.

[40] Atkinson, I, 72, 176-77.

[41] Robert S. Pinals, "How Admiral Rodney's disability saved the American Revolution," *The Pharos*, Spring, 2021.

[42] Pinals.

[43] Pinals.

Part Two:

Doctors Battle for America

CHAPTER TWELVE

DR. BENJAMIN CHURCH COMMITS TREASON, 1775

He hardly fit the mold of a British spy. By the very beginning of the American Revolution, Dr. Benjamin Church had already established himself as a respected Boston physician and a high-profile patriot leader, but within just a few months his life completely unraveled.

Dr. Benjamin Church's fall from grace

Born in 1734 in Newport, Rhode Island, young Benjamin Church moved with his family to Boston, where he followed in the footsteps of many successful men of the town, attending the Boston Latin School and graduating from Harvard College.[1] Church began his studies of medicine as an apprentice and then sailed to England where he received a medical degree from London Medical College. While in London, he married Hannah Hill, an English woman, and the newly-weds returned to Boston upon completion of his medical studies. His reputation both as a skilled physician and patriot blossomed. He was a man of many parts. Benjamin Church wrote poetry and prose and contributed to a patriot newspaper. Before long, he met the political leaders of Boston, John and Sam Adams, John Hancock, and fellow physician Joseph Warren. After the Boston Massacre on March 5,1770, Dr. Church treated the wounded and worked on a committee to protest the massacre to Massachusetts Royal Governor, Thomas Hutchinson. The patriots established an annual oration to commemorate the "bloody tragedy of the Fifth of March," and in recognition of Church's standing and oratorical skills, Dr. Church was selected to give the Boston Massacre commemoration speech in 1773. The next year, he was elected to the Massachusetts Provincial

Congress, the patriots' governing body. Church was appointed a member of the Provincial Congress's Committee of Safety, its executive branch. By 1774, he "enjoyed a position of trust and responsibility just below that occupied by Warren, Hancock, and Sam Adams".[2]

More responsibility awaited Church as the war began. The Continental Congress sought a distinguished doctor to serve as Director-General of the Continental Army Medical Department. Based upon his professional reputation and skills and patriot credentials, Church was appointed as the first Director General with broad powers to inspect the regimental hospitals, examine the regimental surgeons, run the General Hospital, and transfer patients from regimental hospitals to the General Hospital. However, tensions began to mount from the outset. With good reason, Church viewed many regimental surgeons with disdain, considering them poorly qualified and partially trained. And because of his shortage of medications and supplies early in 1775 (due to inadequate Congressional funding), Church could not provide the regimental surgeons with needed stocks, thus earning their anger. Believing that the regimental hospitals were expensive and wasteful, Church wanted them closed with all care delivered by the general hospital. When the problems between the first Director General and the regimental surgeons got to the breaking point, General Washington ordered an inquiry, but the matter died when Church submitted his resignation on September 20, 1775, citing poor health. Despite his short tenure as Director-General, Church still seemed above reproach.

It is uncertain exactly when Dr. Church began corresponding with the British, but he may have begun communicating with Governor Hutchinson and British Commander in Chief General Thomas Gage even before Lexington and Concord (April 1775).[3] But by July 1775, he was certainly providing intelligence to the British. That month, Church wrote a coded letter to British Major Cane (Reiss refers to him as "Major Carne,"[4] including an account of American forces surrounding Boston. In the letter, Church declared his devotion to the Crown and "asked for directions for continuing the correspondence."[5]

Church was a handsome man who maintained a high lifestyle and had a mistress in Boston. His motivation to become a British informer remains speculative, but a good bet was his desire for British gold. Church probably had expenses that were beyond the means of even a successful man of medicine. He had built a large house, and he also had his mistress to support.[6]

Church's ciphered letter was intercepted and made its way to General Washington in September 1775. Washington called a court of inquiry consisting of general officers to investigate. Washington himself decided to preside. Church acknowledged writing the letter but defended himself by claiming that he intended to show the British the great American numbers and strong positions to keep the British from attacking while patriot forces were still actually poorly supplied.[7] He further hoped his letter would end the fighting. The military court of inquiry didn't buy Church's explanation. They found him guilty and referred Church's case to Congress because the American Articles of War at the time had no punishment for treason.[8]

Washington's letter transmitting the case to Congress revealed the circuitous course of Church's coded, treasonous letter. Washington received Church's letter from "one Wainwood, an inhabitant of Newport" who said the letter had been left with him "by a woman who was kept by Doctor Church."[9] She gave Wainwood (Reiss refers to him as "Wormwood")[10] the letter with strict instructions to deliver it to Captain James Wallace of the Royal Navy or two other British officials. Wainwood, suspecting "some improper correspondence, kept the letter and after some time opened it, but not able to read it, laid it up, where it remained until he received an obscure letter from the woman expressing an anxiety as to the original letter." Wainwood then sent the letter through an intermediary in Providence to Washington, who "secured the woman, and she "was at length brought to a confession and named Doctor Church" as the letter's author.

Congress found Church guilty on October 17,1775 and sent him to an underground prison in Norwich, Connecticut "without use of pen, ink and paper, and that no person be allowed to converse with him except in the presence and hearing of a magistrate."[11] In January 1776, he was permitted "considerable movement under guard" because of the ill effects of strict confinement on his health. In May, Church was allowed to return to Massachusetts under bond. For reasons of ill-health at age forty-four years, he was exiled to the West Indies in 1778, but his ship was lost at sea. He was never heard from again.

Church's defenders point out that at the time of his coded correspondence with the British, independence was still a year in the future and that Church viewed himself as wanting to restore good relations between the Mother Country and her North American colonies. But in the view of his American contemporaries, his letter branded him as a traitor to the cause "to which he was ostensibly giving distinguished service."[12]

The Continental Army Medical Department after Church's Treason

Church's treason added new difficulties for the Medical Department on top of the underlying old problems of an ineffective organization, conflicts between the Director-General and the regimental surgeons, and chronic shortages of funds from Congress for medications and supplies. Medical care for the American wounded at Lexington and Concord had been provided by local physicians. The Massachusetts Provincial Congress developed an interim system of care which was taken over by the Continental Congress on July 27, 1775, five and half weeks after the Battle of Bunker Hill.[13] Now, after Church's treachery, the regimental surgeons felt emboldened to defy the

Director-General. Congress had to find the right leader to get the Medical Department on course.

In October 1775, Congress turned to Doctor John Morgan of Philadelphia as the second Director General. (See Chapter Ten for his prior career.) Thus, stepping into the fraught directorship was America's most distinguished physician, but even that distinction did not lead to success. Hard-working, but haughty and perfectionistic, Morgan clashed not only with the regimental surgeons whom he looked down upon, but also with other senior doctors in the Medical Department. Notably, he and Doctor William Shippen, with whom he co-founded the first medical school, had an intense rivalry. Morgan was criticized by Shippen but defended himself claiming that he cared for the sick and wounded surrounding Boston, arranged shipment of medical supplies from Boston to New York in spring 1776, and had excellent stewardship of the limited medical stores. Yet Shippen was joined by Rush in accusing Morgan of confiscating supplies in Boston and withholding medications from regimental surgeons. Morgan rightly believed that Shippen, who had powerful political connections, undercut him. In January 1777, just fifteen months after Morgan assumed the directorship, Congress had enough of the infighting and fired Morgan.

Morgan continued to fight for his reputation, publishing a pamphlet in his defense later in 1777 and collecting letters of support from General Washington and senior officers of the General Hospital. Morgan did not return to the medical faculty but practiced in Philadelphia until his death in October 1781 at fifty-three years of age.

The turbulence continued as Congress appointed Doctor Willam Shippen as the third Medical Director in two years.[14] Shippen came from a prominent Philadelphia family, which included two brothers-in-law in Congress, and married Alice Lee, from an upper-class Virginia family. Like Morgan, he received his MD in Edinburgh. (Please see Chapter Ten for more about his prior career.)

In the interim between Morgan's firing (January 1777) and Shippen's appointment four months later, Shippen had submitted a plan for the re-organization of the medical department. With minor modifications, it was quickly approved by Congress. At last, it seemed that Congress found the right doctor to lead the troubled Medical Department.

However, Shippen got off to a rocky start having to deal with the persisting problems plus accelerating costs. Lacking Morgan's work ethic, Shippen was lax in supervising hospitals under his care. Although Shippen was charming and affable in social settings, in his administrative position, he, like Morgan, wound up quarrelling with other doctors. The director of a hospital in Virginia, Doctor Rickman, complained to Congress that Shippen had usurped his authority. Undercutting Shippen, Congress failed to support their Director-General and backed Rickman.

While Shippen was Director-General, Congress finally cleared Morgan of Shippen's charges of misconduct and inefficiency in July 1779, but Morgan sought vengeance right away by accusing Shippen of malpractice and misconduct, charging Shippen with fraud, improprieties in his accounts, and neglect of duties. Doctor Benjamin Rush, who had joined Shippen in attacks on Morgan, now joined Morgan in attacks on Shippen. The charges resulted in an eventual court-martial of Shippen in spring 1780. Shippen mounted a strong defense including letters from Washington and Benedict Arnold, who at the time was still a glorified American battlefield hero. The third director was acquitted by the narrowest margin—a single vote.[15]

The department was reorganized in October 1780, and as a face-saving measure, Shippen remained director. Yet attacks by Morgan went on unabated, and an exhausted William

Shippen finally resigned in January 1781. After the war, despite the court martial, Shippen returned to his position in Philadelphia society and served in many public roles including President of the College of Physicians. He died in Philadelphia at age 71 years. Thus ended the Medical Department's shameful saga of vitriol, pettiness, and failure of leadership.

For the last two years of the war (during which there was little military action), Congress finally found the correct man to direct the Medical Department.[16] An honorable and skilled physician and administrator, John Cochran was born in 1730, but unlike his three predecessors, did not attend medical school. He got his medical training through an apprenticeship in Lancaster, Pennsylvania, in farming country about seventy miles west of Philadelphia. During the French and Indian War (1754-1763), he served as a surgeon's mate in a British regiment and received great experience guided by the English surgeons. After that war, he gained key political connections by marrying into the Schuyler family, becoming the brother-in-law of Major General Philip Schuyler, who commanded the Continental Army's Northern Department. As part of his practice in New Jersey in the early 1770s, Cochran developed a wide reputation for his skills in smallpox inoculation. In late 1776, he joined Washington's Army during its retreat through New Jersey and was with the army when it famously crossed the Delaware on December 25, 1776. Early the next spring, he achieved administrative recognition by working with Shippen on his plan to reorganize the Medical Department. Based upon his reputation and ties to Shippen, Cochran became Surgeon General of the Middle Department (including Pennsylvania, New Jersey, Maryland, and Delaware) and head of the flying hospital, a mobile care unit of surgeons and assistants to provide prompt care of the wounded on the battlefield. In 1777-78, he cared for the wounded after the Battles of the Brandywine and Germantown and for the sick and injured at Valley Forge.

When Shippen resigned under pressure in 1781, Cochran was the natural selection by Congress as the final Director General. Although he had to deal with many of the entrenched problems, he wisely kept above the fray and competently oversaw the closing of the Medical Department as the war ended officially in September 1783. Afterwards, he left the military and died in 1807 at age seventy-eight years. Cochran never had the formal medical education nor the prominent national reputation of Church, Morgan, and Shippen, but there was not a breath of scandal during his tenure. It is tempting to think how differently the medical department might have accomplished its duties to the health of the troops if Congress had selected Dr. John Cochran in the first place.

Medical Care in the British Army

To gain further insight into the realities of medical care in the Revolutionary War, we now look to the British system. At the outbreak of the Revolutionary War in 1775, England had been fighting in North America for over a century. There was the English Civil War of 1650-1652, the Anglo-Dutch Wars of 1652-1674, the War of Spanish Succession of 1701-1714, and the Seven Years' War of 1756-1763. Accordingly, the English had considerable experience in organizing military medical services for foreign campaigns. However, the British army administration was cumbersome.[17] Further, supporting an army of 30,000 men for war in North America created a host of new problems of nearly unimaginable proportions. Nearly every vial of medicine and every set of surgical instruments had to be purchased in England, shipped 3500 miles to America, and then distributed to where it was needed. It was a Byzantine process.

Overall responsibility for the conduct of the war in North America rested in London with the Secretary at War, a post occupied from 1765 to 1778 by Lord Barrington, and the Secretary of State for the Colonies, occupied by George Germain, First Viscount Sackville, from 1775 to 1785. Advising these secretaries on medical matters in London, was the Inspector-General of Regimental Infirmaries, a position held by the very influential Doctor Robert Adair since 1760.

Serving as the model for the Continental Army, the British Army in North America had both general and regimental hospitals. Prominent physicians were appointed by the Secretary at War to run the general hospitals. Other positions at the general hospitals were purveyors (commissariat officers to purchase and distribute food and medical supplies), staff surgeons (one of whom was selected as Chief surgeon), apothecaries, and hospital mates. At the start of the Revolutionary War, two general hospitals were set up where the British had large numbers of soldiers. In September 1775, the Secretary at War sent instructions from London for the Boston General Hospital and in February 1776, for another general hospital in Quebec.[18,19] From 3500 miles away, Lord Barrington's instructions were exquisitely detailed, even specifying that the senior physician was to attend the sick, prescribe diets and medicines, and keep the wards clean and not crowded. To make communications worse, the London government often aggravated the six to eight weeks it took for instructions and dispatches to cross the Atlantic by delaying replies or orders for weeks. Running a war in North America from London was just too inefficient.

Funds for operating the British general hospitals came in part from the government but also from deductions, called stoppages, from the meager pay of soldiers admitted to a hospital. When a private's daily pay was eight pence, the daily stoppage for a general hospital patient was fully five pence.[20,21] Soldiers who developed wounds, injuries or diseases in service to the crown had to contribute much of their daily pay for their own care.

For the British regimental hospitals, commissions of the surgeon were signed by the commander in chief in North America, but there were no regulations regarding qualifications for appointment. As one Eighteenth-Century British army physician wrote, many became regimental surgeons through "interest and misapplied recommendations" with skills having been "almost none, or at best, extremely limited".[22] The regimental surgeon's station was a lowly one. On returns (which were recurring military reports) of regimental officers, he was placed below the ensigns (the lowest ranking officers). The regimental surgeon's mates' appointments were solely in the hands of the regiment's commanding officer, the colonel. With no regulations for these appointments, Hamilton, a contemporary surgeon, noted that he "could point out cases, where a common soldier from the ranks, after assisting the surgeon of the regiment, in spreading plasters for some time ... was appointed mate thereof".[23] To assist the surgeon and mates, there were orderlies (men from the ranks assigned to the hospital) and nurses (women camp followers hired to work in the hospital).

For care for the rapidly increasing number of soldiers sent to North America in 1776, it was clear that direction could not come solely from London. In early 1777, the Secretary of War appointed an Inspector of Hospitals, but still more supervision was needed. In March 1777, Lord Barrington appointed a distinguished physician, James Napier, to a newly created position of Superintendent-General of Hospitals for His Majesty's Forces in North America. Napier seemed perfectly suited as he had had a similar position in North America during the French and Indian War. With painful delay, it was not until eighteen months later that Barrington proposed sending Napier to America, only to find that Napier declined. The Secretary at War offered the position to Robert Adair, who found himself "not able to quit England." An exasperated Barrington, then appointed Doctor John Mervin Nooth, who was already in America as Purveyor (a military officer responsible for supplying equipment and food), and was thus denied the excuses that Napier and Adair provided. The difficulty in filling this position was most likely based upon officers not wanting to leave the comfort of England, the administrative entanglements of the system, and the developing unpopularity of the war.

Thus, despite a century of fighting North American wars, much of the British Army's medical care was of poor quality even for the standards of the Eighteenth Century. And at the outbreak of the war, care was organized in an antiquated fashion. In part, it was overly centralized with minute details coming from London, but in other ways, it was too decentralized with inadequate supervision of regimental hospitals. Finding the right medical person was fraught with delays and personal issues.

Failure of leadership

In the end, the chaos in the medical directorate of both armies was a failure of leadership. While, secure in their halls and their offices, the American Congress and the London ministers fiddled with their military medical departments, soldiers wearing Continental buff and blue or British scarlet suffered and died.

---

[1] "Surgeons General: Benjamin Church," AMEDD Center of History & Heritage, website.

[2] Reiss, 51-55.

[3] Reiss, 53.

[4] Reiss, 54.

[5] "Surgeons General: Benjamin Church," AMEDD Center of History & Heritage.

[6] Reiss, 53.

[7] "Surgeons General: Benjamin Church," AMEDD Center of History & Heritage.

[8] Reiss, 52.

[9] "Surgeons General: Benjamin Church," AMEDD Center of History & Heritage.

[10] Reiss, 54.

Notes, continued

[11] "Surgeons General: Benjamin Church," AMEDD Center of History & Heritage.

[12] Ibid.

[13] Reiss, 50-51.

[14] Reiss, 61-67.

[15] Reiss, 65-67.

[16] Reiss, 67-70.

[17] Curtis, 50.

[18] Curtis, 22.

[19] Carleton Papers, Vol 1 #54-55 and Vol 4 #364.

[20] Curtis, 22.

[21] Carleton Papers, Vol 1 #54-55 and Vol 4 #364.

[22] Hamilton, 3.

[23] Hamilton, 3.

CHAPTER THIRTEEN

GENERAL (ALSO DOCTOR) HUGH MERCER MAKES THE ULTIMATE SACRIFICE AT PRINCETON, 1777

In his career, Hugh Mercer fought disease at the bedside and the British on the battlefield. Born in Aberdeen, Scotland in 1726 to a Presbyterian minister and his wife, Hugh Mercer received his medical degree from the University of Aberdeen at the age of nineteen years.[1,2] The very next year, he joined the forces of Charles Edward Stuart, called "Bonnie Prince Charlie," in Scotland as an assistant surgeon. The Bonnie Prince was a "spurned pretender" to the British throne and led the Jacobite rebellion to restore the Stuart line to power. The British sent a powerful army to Scotland to crush the uprising and defeated the Stuart army at Culloden Moor in April 1746. Dr. Mercer found himself an immediate fugitive hunted by the British. With the help of family and friends, he managed to escape Scotland by sailing to America. Mercer arrived in Philadelphia in May 1747 and was quickly able to set up his medical practice in Pennsylvania, near present day Mercersburg, named for him. When the French and Indian War broke out, he served now on the British side, but as captain in a Pennsylvania militia company, not as a physician. On September 8, 1756, while on a raid against Shawnee and Delaware Indians in Western Pennsylvania, Mercer was severely wounded and got separated from his company. He managed to survive two weeks alone in the wilderness before reaching safety at Fort Littleton. A newspaper account in late September heroized his "miraculous escape." Mercer lived "ten Days on two dried Clams and a Rattle snake, with the Assistance of a few Berries. The Snake kept sweet for several Days, and, coming near Fort Shirley, he found a Piece of dry Beef, which our People had lost, and on Trial rejected it, because the Snake was better. His wounded Arm is in a good Way, thou' it could be but badly drest, and a Bone broken."[3]

After his illustrious service during the French and Indian War, he moved to Fredericksburg, Virginia, where he was a successful physician and apothecary. A patient in 1771 was George Washington's mother, Mary Ball Washington, who was treated with bleeding, blistering plasters, purges and vomiting for an "unspecified illness".[4] In Fredericksburg, he married Isabella Gordon, with whom he had five children.

At the outset of the Revolutionary War in 1775, Mercer became a line officer, appointed colonel of the Third Virginia Regiment. By June 1776, Washington appointed him brigadier general in the Continental Army and commander of the Flying Camp, made up mainly of militia as a rapid response unit to defend New Jersey during the campaign in New York in August through November 1776. Mercer found that this command severely tested his patience because of the "reluctant, often disobedient, militiamen."[5] In mid-November, as Washington began his retreat westward across New Jersey, the Flying Camp was disbanded. Mercer was given a new command and fought valiantly at Trenton. Ten days later, at the Battle of Princeton on January 3, 1777, Mercer was leading the American vanguard when attacked by a much larger British force. He rallied his men, but his horse was shot out from under him. Mercer became separated from his men but continued to fight while dismounted. Even though British troops surrounded him, he refused to surrender. Hugh Mercer had had a lifetime of close calls, but fate now caught up with him. He was wounded in the head and body with seven bayonet stabbings. He was taken from the battlefield to the nearby Clark House (which still stands) where he was attended by Dr. Benjamin Rush, who came from Philadelphia to see him. However, it was known that Mercer's bayonet wounds were fatal. He lingered for nine agonizing days before succumbing to his injuries on January 12, 1777. Mercer's remains were removed for burial in Philadelphia. Dr. Benjamin Rush wrote of Mercer, "A fine companion, a sincere friend, a true patriot, and a brave general".[6] John Trumball's 1789 painting, *The Death of General Mercer at the Battle of Princeton, January 3, 1777,* immortalizes him.

By coincidence, also on the Princeton battlefield was another physician-warrior, Colonel John Haslet (1727-1777), a native of Ireland, an ordained a Presbyterian minister, and a Glasgow-educated physician. He migrated to America and, after service in the Pennsylvania militia in the French and Indian War, moved to Milford, Delaware. In 1776, Haslet was in command of the Delaware First Continental Regiment and, like Mercer, fought throughout the New York campaign. By a tragic twist of fate, Haslet died next to Mercer when hit by a British bullet.

Before and After Princeton

Eighteen months before Mercer's death, another physician-warrior met death on the battlefield and was also immortalized in a John Trumball painting completed in 1786. Doctor Joseph Warren, recently described as "the Revolution's Lost Hero",[7] was an esteemed Boston physician from a long line of Massachusetts doctors. He learned medicine as an apprentice. In 1775, Warren was a thirty-four-year-old widower with four young children. A prominent leader in the cause of independence, he was chairman of the Committee of Safety and President of the Massachusetts Provincial Congress. In April 1775, Warren ordered the local militia to form in Lexington and Concord to meet the British Army column sent to capture Samuel Adams and John Hancock and to destroy American military supplies. Two months later at Breed's (Bunker's) Hill in Charlestown (now part of Boston), Warren was one of the American commanders, serving as major general. When the British troops finally took the American fortifications on their third attempt, Warren continued to fight valiantly rather than retreat. He was stabbed repeatedly and died heroically on the field of battle.

Finally, we must take a detour veering strictly from physician-warriors to a former "health care professional" (in today's terms) who became the most infamous traitor in American history. Benedict Arnold began his career as a successful apothecary in Connecticut and early in the Revolutionary War was the boldest battlefield commander in the Continental Army. He led his "men through peril, on land or otherwise, with ferocity, prudence, judgement, luck, and implacable will".[8] Born in 1741 in Connecticut, he served in the French and Indian War as a sixteen-year-old. He then became a pharmacy apprentice to his two older brothers. Five years later, with support from the family, he set up his own firm in New Haven selling medications, surgical instruments, and books.

Arnold's spectacular battlefield record began in the first months of the Revolutionary War. In May 1775, along with Ethan Allen, he seized Fort Ticonderoga from the British. In fall 1775, he led the expedition through the Maine woods to Canada, and in December he was seriously wounded during the heroic attack on Quebec. (See Chapter One.) He recovered, and in autumn 1776 he led a squadron that turned back the invading British fleet on Lake Champlain. The next year at Saratoga, he was again wounded, this time in the leg while leading an attack that turned the critical battle in favor of the Americans. In June 1778, after the British evacuated Philadelphia, Washington made him military governor of the city. While there, as a widower, he married his second wife, Peggy Shippen, of a distinguished Loyalist family and a grandniece of Dr. William Shippen.

However, there was a dark side to Arnold. Described by a contemporary, as hot and impetuous, he feuded with other officers and was investigated by Congress over charges of oppressive behavior while in command of Philadelphia. In early 1780, he was cleared, but his reputation was adversely affected.

He was passed over for promotion to Major General. Arnold attempted to resign his commission but eventually was given command of the fortifications guarding the Hudson River at West Point, New York.[9] At this time, having almost lost his leg to an enemy bullet, having suffered financially during the war, and feeling slighted by other officers and by Congress, he put his "own interests ahead of [his] newborn country's."[10]

In 1780, Arnold secretly began negotiating with the British for their capture of West Point, but in September, the plot was uncovered when Major John Andre, the chief British intelligence officer, was captured with documents revealing Arnold's betrayal. When Arnold got word of Andre's capture, he immediately fled West Point on horseback and escaped to a British ship in the Hudson River. The complete turncoat, Arnold then served as an officer in the British Army in North America. He and his family eventually made it to England where he died in 1801. Washington, always a man of impeccable honor, called Arnold's actions, "Treason of the blackest dye.".[11] Even today, the name of Benedict Arnold remains synonymous with treason.

---

[1] American Battlefield Trust, "Hugh Mercer," accessed December 18, 2025, battlefields.org website.

[2] Crossroads of the American Revolution, "Hugh Mercer Full Biography," revolutionarynj.org/people_biography/hugh-mercer-full-biography/ website.

[3] Crossroads.

[4] Parascondola.

[5] Crossroads.

[6] Atkinson, I, 550.

[7] di Spigna.

[8] Atkinson, I, 428, 552.

[9] Katie Uva. "Benedict Arnold", In *The Digital Encyclopedia of George Washington*, accessed Dec 18, 2025. www.mountvernon.org/library/digitalhistory/digital-encyclopedia/article/benedict-arnold.

Notes, continued

[10] Philbrick, 206, 322.

[11] "Benedict Arnold", MountVernon.org website.

CHAPTER FOURTEEN

DR. JOSIAH BARTLETT SIGNS THE DECLARATION OF INDEPENDENCE, 1776

It is striking that five of the fifty-six signers—nearly ten percent—of the Declaration of Independence were physicians considering that physicians made up only one-tenth of one percent of the colonial population. One historian emphasized that medicine in Eighteenth Century North America did not rank with the law or ministry in either remuneration or prestige and that physicians often sought service in government to improve their reputation and condition. Another historian attributed physicians' support for the revolutionary cause because they believed, as scientists of the day, in the Enlightenment principle of a just society.[1]

In Chapter Thirteen, we saw how Doctors Hugh Mercer, John Haslet, and Joseph Warren exemplified qualities of great leadership beyond their practices as battlefield heroes. Here we will see how the five physician-signers of the Declaration of Independence exhibited great leadership beyond their practices as builders of their states and the nation. Benjamin Rush was the most noted physician-signer, but fans of television political drama may surprisingly recognize another name. Revolutionary-era Doctor Josiah Bartlett (1729-1795) had a fictional namesake almost 250 years later in the critically acclaimed show, *The West Wing* (1999-2006), in which President Josiah "Jed" Bartlet was portrayed by actor Martin Sheen as a direct descendant of physician-signer Josiah Bartlett. (Note that the Eighteenth-Century Bartlett is spelled with two t's while the television Bartlet has one t.)

The real Josiah Bartlett had a long and prominent career in public service as well as in medicine. He was born in

Amesbury, Massachusetts in 1729 to a family of modest means. His writings show that he received a solid boyhood education, but he could not afford to attend college. Attracted to medicine, he was an apprentice under Dr. Nehemiah Ordway, a relative practicing in Amesbury. At the bedside with Dr. Ordway and in his mentor's library, Bartlett studied medicine for six years. At age twenty-one, young Dr. Bartlett established a successful medical practice. The town of Kingston, New Hampshire, with a population of less than 1000, needed a doctor. Another young physician arrived at the same time, but Bartlett's skills attracted the town's attention. He became Kingston's doctor.[2] Bartlett was an innovative doctor. In 1752, when he suffered a raging fever, he successfully used cooling drinks (a cider) for himself, rather than the prevailing use of hot beverages to treat fever. Two years later, he may have also been the first doctor in the area to use Peruvian bark to treat a fever.[3]

From the sole portrait of Bartlett, he appears to have been physically strong, with a firm New England countenance.[4] Likely the town's most eligible bachelor, he married a cousin, Mary Bartlett, in 1754. Mary had a strong character herself and pursued Josiah. By one account, "on a stormy night, Mary knocked on Josiah's door imploring him to visit a sick relative. She then led him to an abandoned farmhouse where she laughed playfully at his gullibility and irritation".[5] The account does not explain what happened immediately thereafter. During their marriage, they had ten children, two of whom died in infancy—a family tragedy common in an era of high childhood mortality.

As Bartlett's practice grew in the 1760s, he trained two apprentice physicians. One apprentice, as it commonly happened, was a relative, his nephew Joseph Bartlett, who went on to practice for many years in Salisbury, sixty miles away. The other apprentice was Amos Gale, who became Bartlett's medical partner and life-long friend. Linking the families even closer, one of the Bartlett daughters married Amos Gale's son, Dr. Amos Gale, Jr.

Josiah Bartlett's extraordinary public career began in 1765 with his election to the New Hampshire General Assembly. Over the next decade, as tensions with England mounted, he spent more time on political matters and less time in Kingston on his practice. The first Provincial Congress of New Hampshire elected Bartlett a delegate to the First Continental Congress meeting in Philadelphia in 1774. However, he could not travel to Pennsylvania because he was overseeing the reconstruction of the family house which had been destroyed by fire in 1774. In August 1775, Bartlett was reappointed to the Continental Congress. On September 5, he and his fellow delegate John Langdon left New Hampshire for Philadelphia. The 350-mile journey took them eleven days.

When he arrived in the capital, there was an outbreak of smallpox. Having had neither the natural disease nor the inoculation, he went to fellow delegate Dr. Benjamin Rush to get inoculated. In a letter to his wife on October 2, 1775, Bartlett described his own experience. "I Can now with pleasure inform you that I have been Inoculated for the Small Pox and am almost Got well of it. I had it very favorable not about 20 pock or thereabout tho I was Confined by the fever to the House 5 or 6 Days."[6]

Bartlett served a total of nineteen months in Congress (September 1775-March 1776, May-November 1776, and May-November 1778), where he was a political moderate with high moral principles. In spring 1776, he was appointed to the congressional committee that drafted the Articles of Confederation. The basic Articles of Confederation were drafted during the summer of 1776, but the articles themselves were not finally ratified until 1781. Although Bartlett and others favored a strong central government, the articles wound up creating a weak one leaving most power with the states. Having witnessed the consequences of the British government, most members of Congress feared the creation of a powerful central government in the new United States. Chief features of the articles included the absence of an executive branch and very limited ability to tax.[7]

While the articles were being drafted, another committee was preparing a declaration of independence for the colonies. In June 1776, not all delegates to the Continental Congress favored that course, but Bartlett did. On June 3rd, he wrote to his wife, "I hope ... that kind providence will give us success & victory that the wickedness and villainy of our enemies will fall on their own heads, and that America may be for ever separated from the tyranny of Britain."[8] The Declaration of Independence was approved by Congress, and on July 4, 1776 Bartlett signed the copy along with William Whipple for New Hampshire. On July 15th, Bartlett wrote to John Langdon, "The Unparalleled conduct of our Enemies have united the Colonies more firmly than ever."[9]

With no executive branch, the only way Congress could administer the government was through numerous committees. These committees sometimes met in the mornings before the main Congress session, but more often met in evenings, commonly in a tavern. The evening sessions sometimes did not end until midnight. Bartlett served on several committees, notably the Marine Committee and the Secret Committee of Correspondence, which was organized to coordinate diplomatic functions and public relations early in war. During his many months in Congress, Bartlett was well respected and angered few, if any, colleagues. He was honorable with "well-founded principles and upright morals."[10]

Bartlett was back in New Hampshire in 1777 when British General Burgoyne's invading army was advancing down the Lake Champlain-Lake George-Hudson River axis. Learning of a stock of badly needed horses and supplies in Bennington, Vermont, Burgoyne sent a combined British-German force, under Hessian

Lt. Colonel Frederich Baum, to get the supplies. American militia, including units from New Hampshire, rallied to meet Baum's force. Dr. Bartlett and Dr. Nathaneal Peabody accompanied the New Hampshire troops. Numbering over 1000, the American militia surrounded and attacked Baum's men on August 16, 1777, outside Bennington. Responding to the rallying cry of their commander, General John Stark, hero of Bunker Hill, the militia resoundingly defeated the enemy, killing or wounding over 200 and taking 700 prisoners. American casualties were no more than seventy. Drs. Bartlett and Peabody attended the wounded of both sides. The Battle of Bennington weakened Burgoyne's invading force and set the stage for his surrender at Saratoga two months later.

After his last service in Congress in November 1778, Bartlett returned to New Hampshire where he seemed to serve in almost every capacity. He continued his medical practice and also served as justice of the peace, member of the Committee of Safety, and county judge. In 1789, he was commissioned as chief justice of the New Hampshire Superior Court, and in 1790, he was elected president of New Hampshire (the forerunner of governor). In 1788, he was gratified by his state's ratification of the United States Constitution. Finally, in 1792, when New Hampshire adopted a new state constitution, creating a governor as the state's chief executive, Bartlett was elected governor for two consecutive one-year terms.

With continued devotion to medical practice, he established the New Hampshire Medical Society in 1791 and served as its president. He was a far-sighted advocate for high quality care. In a letter to the medical society in 1793, he wrote, "The Practice of Medicine in this State ... might be put under better regulations ... [and] the New Hampshire Medical Society will produce effects greatly beneficial to the community by encouraging Genius & learning in the Medical Science and discouraging ignorant & bold pretenders from practicing an Art which they have no knowledge."[11]

While governor, Bartlett's health began to fail, and he retired from public service in June 1794. He put his will and accounts in order over the next few months. He died at age sixty-six years, in Kingston, his wife having pre-deceased him in 1789.[12] Bartlett left behind a legacy of service to New Hampshire and to the young United States and in a lasting way to the high standards of practice of medicine.

Other physician-signers

Lyman Hall (1724-1790) had the most mysterious career of the physician-signers. Born in New England, he graduated from Yale and became a Congregational minister in Fairfield, Connecticut. Two years later, he ran into trouble when he was charged with "immoral conduct."[13] After a hearing, he was dismissed from his pastorate. The tantalizing, full story shall never be known as the records of his hearing were burned when the British torched many Fairfield buildings in 1779. Perhaps because of persuasive repentance, he was restored in good standing as a minister. In 1752, he married, but his first wife died just thirteen months afterward. Hall soon remarried and had one son who died at the age of twenty-seven. With all the turmoil, Hall found the ministry "unrewarding" and took an apprenticeship under a Fairfield physician. In 1756, for unknown reasons, he moved south winding up in Georgia, where he had a rice plantation, owned enslaved persons, and established a bustling medical practice. He also became active in patriot meetings. Georgia, the newest colony, was the only one that did not send delegates to the First Continental Congress in 1774. When Georgia finally sent delegates to the Second Continental Congress in March 1775, Dr. Hall went to Philadelphia along with two fellow delegates. In Philadelphia, Hall played a retiring role in the debates but was active in crucial committee work. Fittingly, his work addressed medication supply and care of the sick and wounded. His last day in Congress was in February 1777. Returning to Georgia, Lyman Hall, now a steady, mild-mannered physician, became the state's governor in 1783. Like Bartlett, he died at age sixty-six.

Yet another New Englander, Oliver Wolcott (1725-1797) was born with a silver spoon in his mouth, the son of the Connecticut Deputy Governor for the Crown. He was a classmate at Yale of Lyman Hall. Deciding on a medical career, Wolcott became an apprentice physician for two years under his much older brother. However, by 1751, he gave up medicine and entered political service. Initially, he was a county high sheriff. In 1755, he married and had five children, one of whom died in infancy. As the revolution heated up, Wolcott, described as "clear-minded and independent",[14] was appointed to represent Connecticut in the Continental Congress and arrived in January 1776. Wolcott was a Whig politically and brought "broad experience, solid intelligence, and nationalistic sympathies"[15] to his extensive committee work dealing with commerce, maritime affairs, Indian affairs, and the treasury. Wolcott's service in Congress was interrupted in late June 1776 by a severe illness, requiring him to leave Philadelphia. He was absent at the original signing of the Declaration of Independence on July 2, 1776, but was allowed to sign in October when he returned to Philadelphia. During the war, the Connecticut government elected him a brigadier general in the state militia. He led a force of 300 men to Upstate New York and saw action at the critical battle at Saratoga on October 7,1777. A man of "rugged common sense and exceptional integrity," Wolcott served after the war as Commissioner of Indian Affairs and as Lieutenant Governor of Connecticut. He died at age of seventy-two.

Finally, Matthew Thornton (1714-1803) was born in Ireland and moved with his family to New Hampshire, where he was educated and served his medical apprenticeship under Dr. Thomas Green. Green himself had a colorful story as he had apprenticed under two English surgeons who had been "outlawed, as pirates and who boarded with" Thorton's father for several years.[16] Thorton's practice blossomed, and he was able to purchase land from which he drew substantial additional income. In 1745, during King George's War (also called the War of Austrian Succession in Europe), he was an under-surgeon in a military expedition to Louisburg, Canada. He did not marry until he was forty-six and chose a bride who was twenty-eight years younger. She bore five children, all of whom survived to adulthood. Thorton began his public career at age forty and served in the Provincial Assembly and as a county judge. In 1770, at age fifty-six years, he was commissioned colonel in a New Hampshire militia regiment but saw no action in the Revolutionary War. Thorton was sixty when the war began. He was selected by New Hampshire as a delegate to Congress in 1776. Even though he arrived after July 1776, he was permitted to sign the Declaration of Independence in November 1776. Impeccably honest and good humored, Thorton "abounded in anecdotes".[17] Arriving in Philadelphia, he like Dr. Bartlett took the smallpox inoculation and paid the doctor his bill of 18 dollars. His work in Congress was modest as he served only on a few lesser committees. He left Philadelphia in May 1777 having written home that "my constitution will not allow my staying here longer".[18] After the revolution, he retired from medical practice and died suddenly in June 1803 at age of eighty-nine years. He had accumulated a sizeable estate valued at $24,000 when an acre of farmland cost four dollars and a pewter basin twenty-five cents.[19]

Doctors Bartlett, Hall, Wolcott, and Thorton are lesser-known physician-signers than Benjamin Rush. All had New England roots. None of the four attended medical school but, like most physicians at the time, learned medicine as apprentices. Though nearly forgotten by history, they were all dedicated and successful public servants at a time when their country desperately needed their skills and leadership. In this chapter, we have explored the lives of physicians in treating patients and in founding the country. In the years during and immediately after the revolution, these physicians took on the burden of creating a politically visionary society, one unlike the world had ever seen before.

---

[1] Gifford, 3.

[2] Gifford, 99.

[3] Gifford, 100.

[4] Ibid., 111.

[5] Ibid., 103.

[6] Ibid., 104.

[7] The Articles of Confederation proved fatally flawed leading to the Constitution of the United States, drafted in 1787 and ratified in 1788.

[8] Gifford, 107.

[9] Gifford, 108.

[10] Ibid., 112.

[11] Ibid., 117.

[12] Ibid., 114, 118.

[13] Gifford., 125.

[14] Gifford, 54.

[15] Ibid.

[16] Ibid., 71.

[17] Gifford, 82-83.

[18] Ibid., 87.

[19] Ibid., 88-89.

ACKNOWLEDGEMENTS

Just over a year ago, I was in the midst of writing a third historical novel, the sequel to the two set in the American Revolution that I had published in 2020 and 2024. Then, knowing the United States was beginning its celebration of 250 years of independence, I pivoted from the world of fiction. I had already given a series of lectures on medicine in the American Revolution and thought it would be a quick project to develop a book on the subject. It was one of those many times in my life that I fooled myself. As I began to write, I researched numerous additional sources, but my first version read like a heavy medical textbook. I wanted to tell the great story not just for physicians but mainly for a wide range or readers interested in America's founding. Once again, I turned to Amy Benedicty as both an editor and friend. With her insightful direction, we completely revised the book emphasizing the personal stories as well as the facts. I am indebted for her critical views of the book's organization as well as her exquisite attention to detail as we read every line aloud. I am incredibly thankful for her expertise and dedication in working with me to forge the final product. For her creativity in design, I thank my friend Judith Lippe once again. She researched many ideas to come up with the imaginative and captivating cover. For his many talents and patience, I thank my friend Howard Bomze, who worked creatively with Judith Lippe on the design of the book cover, helped select the illustrations and for his completeness and attention to detail in preparing and uploading the final manuscript for publication on Amazon. I also express my thanks to Madeline Gunther, who carefully finalized the manuscript assuring that all the i's were dotted and the t's were crossed.

During the preparation of the work, I relied upon numerous colleagues and friends and want to thank Drs. Roger Newman, Dave Davis, and Gary Siegel, Suzanne and Darragh

Howard, and Albert Sukoff. Rich Melnicoff once again provided strategies for marketing and tracking, and Stuart Gibbs provided exceedingly helpful insight and commentary at many stages on the writing. Greta Alexander gave me valued ideas as the book developed and brought renewed joy and sunshine into my life. I am indebted to have so talented a group of friends and so incredible a family who bring a world of love, pride and happiness.

APPENDICES

Appendix A. A descriptive chronology of the American Revolutionary War

The American Revolutionary War began on April 19,1775 and ended eight years and five months later, on September 3,1783 with the signing of the Treaty of Paris. It was the longest war in the country's history until the 2003-2011 Iraq War, which was four months longer. About 7,000 American and 2,000 French troops were killed in battle and several times these numbers were wounded. Of the King's troops, about 8,000 British, 1,200 Germans, and 1,700 Loyalists were killed.[1] In the war at sea, the toll for the Royal Navy was 1,240 seaman killed in action but 18,500 dead from disease.[2]

Most killed and wounded on both sides were rank and file soldiers—for plain reasons. There were a lot more of them, and they were more often in the direct line of fire. Yet, senior officers made the ultimate sacrifice as well. In Chapter Twelve, we read of the deaths in battle of three physician-warriors: Brigadier General Hugh Mercer and Colonel John Haslett at Princeton and Major General Joseph Warren at Bunker Hill. Among other American officers, Major General Richard Montgomery died of wounds in the attack on Quebec (December 1776). American Brigadier General Benedict Arnold was seriously wounded at the same battle and then again at Saratoga (October 1777). Washington's aide, The Marquis de Lafayette, was wounded in the leg at Brandywine (September 1777), and Brigadier General Nicolas Herkimer, commander of the county militia in Upstate New York, died from a leg wound at the Battle of Oriskany (August 1777).[3] And American Brigadier General Casmir Pulaski died of gangrene complicating a wound of his pelvis at Savannah (October 1779).[4] Washington was thrilled by battle and often led from the front. He came within easy range of enemy fire once trying to form the militia at Kip's Bay on Manhattan

(September1776) and again rallying the troops at Princeton (January 1777) and also scouting prior to Brandywine (September 1777). Yet, he was never wounded, nor were any of his senior staff, Nathaneal Greene, John Sullivan, Horatio Gates, or Charles Lee, despite being in the thick of battle.

After a decade of political struggle about colonial rights, taxes and trade, the war broke out in Lexington and Concord, Massachusetts, with the "shot heard round the world." On that fateful day in April 1775, the British sent 700 men to arrest patriot leaders, Sam Adams and John Hancock, in Lexington and then destroy American arms in Concord, nineteen miles from Boston. In Lexington, the British regiments and town militia faced each other in typical parallel lines on the town green. It is not known which side fired the first shot, but a skirmish ensued, leaving several American dead and wounded. Adams and Hancock had already escaped. The British marched an additional seven miles to Concord, where they found preciously few colonial arms, exchanged fire with the local militia across Concord Bridge, and then began their march back to Boston, having achieved neither of their objectives. Now the countryside was alarmed, and thousands of New England militia assaulted the redcoat column by firing upon them from behind trees and rocks. The American tactic gave them a one-sided advantage. As shown in the table, the total American dead and wounded amounted to about ninety men, but the British suffered 246 killed and wounded, nearly a third of the original number marching from Boston.

For the next two months, the British hunkered down in Boston, surrounded by thousands of militiamen. On June 17th, the British awoke to find that the Americans had fortified Breed's Hill (commonly mis-identified as its neighboring mound, Bunker Hill), and American cannons threatened them in the town. The British commander, General William Howe, ordered an immediate attack to dislodge the militia. Forming in traditional linear array, the redcoats marched shoulder to shoulder up the hill toward the American earthen fortifications—into withering

American musket fire. Only on their third attempt—when American ammunition ran out—were the British able to take the hilltop fortification, but at great cost. Owing to the tactics, this was a bloody battle. American casualties totaled over 400, but British amounted to over 1,000. The toll was so heavy, including all the British commander's staff except him, that he subsequently avoided frontal, linear array attacks in almost every battle.

General George Washington soon arrived in Boston as commander in chief. A stalemate developed over the winter, but in the March Washington took advantage of a British oversight. He fortified Dorchester Heights overlooking Boston from the south. From this position, American cannons again threatened the British Army, which had no choice but to evacuate Boston. On March 17, 1776, the British army, along with thousands of loyalists, sailed from Boston to Halifax, Nova Scotia, but fully intent on returning to their colonies to crush the rebellion.

While the Americans surrounded the British in Boston in 1775, a band of 1,300 Americans left New England in a heroic effort to invade Canada, certain it would become the fourteenth state. Trekking through over 200 miles of Maine wilderness in bitter late fall weather and suffering from starvation and smallpox, they emerged six weeks later before the citadel of Quebec. They were joined by General Montgomery's troops who had just taken Montreal. With the Canadians having no desire to join the rebellion, the Americans attacked the small British detachment and the Canadian militia inside the walled city during a late December blizzard. The attack was easily repulsed, forcing the Americans to lay siege to Quebec through the brutal Canadian winter. In May, when a relieving British force sailed up the St. Lawrence River, the haggard American Army retreated to New York. The American attempt in Canada ended in complete failure. American killed and wounded numbered about 60, but over 400 were captured. On the other hand, British and Canadian loses were only six dead and nineteen wounded.

Table. Killed and Wounded for American* and King's Forces* in Selected Battles

Battle, Year	American Killed	American Wounded	King's Forces	King's Forces
Lexington & Concord, Massachusetts, April	50	39	73	174
Breed's (Bunker's) Hill, Massachusetts,	140	271	226	828
Charleston, South Carolina, June 1776	12	28	91	170
Long Island (Brooklyn), New York,	**	**	64	291
White Plains, New York, October 1776	50-150	>150	48	182
Trenton, New Jersey, December 1776	2	4	22	92
Brandywine, Pennsylvania,	250	600	93	488
Germantown, Pennsylvania,	182	521	71	448
Saratoga, 1777	90	240	440	695, plus 6,200
Guilford Court House, North Carolina, March	79	185	93	413
Yorktown, Virginia, October 1781	8	301	142-309	326-595

Note on sources: Reports of casualties were unreliable and sometimes conflicting. I used listings from The American Battlefield Trust.[5]

* French casualties are included in American for Yorktown. German and Loyalist casualties are included for King's Forces.

** Estimates vary, but best ones list 200 Americans killed or wounded plus 900 captured.

By summer 1776, reinforced British forces were eager to end the rebellion. Their target was New York City. The Americans had already figured that out and had begun fortifying the city as early as April. With the aid of thousands of German mercenaries, the British stormed into New York from the sea, with huge fleets from Nova Scotia and the British Isles. Washington had fatefully divided his troops, keeping about half on Manhattan and placing the rest across the East River, in defensive positions in Brooklyn on Long Island. In late August, the British attacked the Brooklyn position first, but learning the lesson from Bunker Hill, they used a flanking march, rather than a frontal attack. This tactic caught the Americans totally by surprise and resulted in a resounding British victory with relatively few British casualties. The Americans suffered heavily including large numbers who were captured. Two weeks later, the British invaded Manhattan at Kip's Bay (today's 34th Street at the East River), over-whelmed a thin American defensive line there, and caused the Americans to retreat in panic to upper Manhattan. General Washington charged from his headquarters in Harlem Heights in upper Manhattan to rally the fleeing Americans retreating from Kip's Bay. It was then that he came within a hundred yards of approaching British rangers and was in immediate danger of being shot. His efforts were to no avail.

Stalemate ensued for a few weeks, with the Americans fortifying Harlem Heights in upper Manhattan and the British occupying the rest of the island. In October, once again, rather than attacking the American defenses in upper Manhattan frontally, the British carried out a flanking attack, this time by a water-borne route, forcing the Americans to evacuate Manhattan. Washington's forces retreated twenty-five miles north of New York City to White Plains, where they constructed a strong, hilltop defensive position. To dislodge the Americans, the British formed in linear array but attacked against the American flank.

Outmaneuvered, the American army sustained over 300 casualties and had to retreat again, this time across New Jersey, staying just ahead of the pursing enemy. Washington's army just made it to the safety of Pennsylvania, across the Delaware River. With his army defeated time and again and dwindled from 20,000 in the summer to just 2500 by late December,

Washington faced a cause-ending crisis. However, he relied upon his bold instincts and risked it all. On Christmas night 1776, he famously crossed the Delaware River into New Jersey and surprised and defeated isolated, sleepy German regiments in Trenton. It was a desperately needed and one-sided victory for the Americans. Ten days later, Washington was victorious over British regiments in Princeton, New Jersey. These two small, but important victories were noted throughout the Americas and in London and Paris; they saved the cause of independence.

While the war was unfolding in the north, the British sent a fleet to capture Charleston, South Carolina thinking loyalist support there would help the royal cause. However, the Carolina militia was anything but loyal to the king. When the British sailed into Charleston harbor, it met with disaster, the result of low tides and devastating American cannon fire. The vaunted Royal Navy was humiliated and limped back to New York. This stunning American victory held the South until the British returned four years later.

For 1777, the British embarked on a two-pronged strategy. The main army left New York on a sea-borne route to capture the American capital, Philadelphia. By traditional European thinking, that should have ended the rebellion. At the same time, a second British invading force stuck from Canada, down the Lake Champlain-Lake George-Hudson River route to separate the New England colonies from the Middle Colonies. With these two armies not able to support each other, the British strategy ended in disaster.

In the Philadelphia campaign, the main British army dealt two severe blows to Washington's main American force. The British routed the Americans at the Battle of the Brandywine in September. It was the largest single day battle of the war with 30,000 soldiers total on both sides. Once again avoiding a frontal attack against established American defenses, the British used a flanking march (like the attack on Long Island the previous

August). The killed and wounded on both sides totaled over 1,300 men. Washington's army was able to escape thanks to a heroic rearguard defense.

Two weeks later, the British marched into Philadelphia without firing a shot. Yet, Washington was not done and attacked the British position in Germantown, outside the American capital, in early October. Although it began well for the Americans, Washington's plan was too complicated, and heavy fog caused delays and confusion. The British had time to regroup and then sent the Americans reeling. American losses included 700 killed and wounded and over 400 captured. However, these two British victories in Pennsylvania were all for naught. Washington's army remained intact, surviving the brutal winter of 1777-1778 at Valley Forge, and after just eight months the British evacuated Philadelphia in spring 1778 to consolidate in New York in the event of a French attack.

The real British calamity occurred that fall in upstate New York, where their invading army became trapped by a huge American force. After two large battles that fall, the invading British army surrendered in entirety (over 6,300) in October 1777 at Saratoga, New York. American casualties numbered about 330 but were light compared with the British and German total of over 1,000 killed and wounded. This American victory was the turning point of the war as the French Alliance followed suit. The French, age-old enemies of the English, had lost Canada at the end of the French and Indian War in the 1760s and were thirsting for revenge. Once they saw a possibility of American military success, they openly jumped in with men, arms, ships, medicines, other supplies, and money.

In 1779, the British again turned their war efforts to the South, still hoping to capitalize on loyalist support. After an easy victory at Savannah, Georgia (October 1779) and capture of Charleston, South Carolina (May 1780), the British turned north into the Carolinas and Virginia where they were met by a resourceful American army, under command of General Nathaneal Greene, Washington's favorite. In a series of battles, Greene wore down the British. At the Battle of Guilford Court House in North Carolina (March 1781), Greene chose a strong defensive position to receive the frontal attack by the British. Greene wisely left the field to the British, but only after inflicting heavy casualties on the British (twice as many as the Americans sustained). Not able to replace their losses and worn down by disease, the British eventually marched into the small port town of Yorktown, Virginia on Chesapeake Bay to rest and await relief from a British fleet from New York. Now, in the summer and fall of 1781, the French alliance paid off handsomely for the Americans. A French fleet was already in American waters and got into Chesapeake Bay before the British ships could. In the naval battle that followed, the French drove off the Royal Navy ships, leaving the British Army in Yorktown isolated. A combined Franco-American Army laid siege to the British positions. With no help of rescue and sustaining hundreds of killed and wounded from devastating cannon fire, the British commander surrendered in October 1781. This was the second British disaster of the war, the surrender of an entire army.

The British government had had enough. The fighting war was basically over, and protracted negotiations ensued, producing the Treaty of Paris two years later. The United States had won its independence.

England, one of the great powers of the era, squandered its best opportunities and lost its American colonies. They sent the wrong generals and had the wrong strategy. Time and distance further hindered the British execution of the war. For the Americans, no one thought they had a chance at the outset, but they eventually developed the right strategy and stayed with the right leader in George Washington.

---

[1] American Revolution Facts, website.

[2] Atkinson, II, 330.

[3] Atkinson, II, 103.

[4] Atkinson, II, 552.

[5] American Battlefield Trust, website, data from listings under individual battles.

Appendix B. Detailed descriptions of surgical procedures

For the reader with an interest in the details of additional Eighteenth Century military surgical operations, I have included the descriptions below. Surgery to treat gunshot wounds is described fully in Chapter Six.

Trephining, also known as trepanning

Known since prehistoric times, trephining is an operation to remove a disc of skull bone. In the Eighteenth Century, surgeons used it relieve pressure on the brain after head wounds or trauma. The operation was carried out with the patient sitting erect in a chair, his head either held firmly by padded, wooden side pieces or by the hands of an assistant. Imagine a regimental surgeon performing trephining on a lieutenant who had been shot in his skull. The surgeon cuts into the skin and tendon with a scalpel and extends the incision at the determined scalp location for the trepanning. Because of brain damage at the site of the head wound, the trephining site is usually a few inches away. The trephine has a bone handle which is affixed to a three-inch long steel shaft. At the other end is a cylindrical saw, three-fourths of an inch in diameter. The surgeon places the teeth of the trephine against the skull and bears down into the bone with twisting pressure. After a half-dozen twists, the surgeon withdraws the instrument to clean bone spicules from the cutting edges. He then replaces the trephine in its track and carefully cuts the rest of the way through the skull. With forceps, he removes the disc of bone from the lieutenant's skull. Through the opening in the skull bone, the surgeon sees the dura mater, the membrane lining the brain. Because of brain hemorrhage, the dura mater bulges, and below it there is dark reddish-black fluid. To conclude the case, the surgeon's assistant fills the trepanned hole with lint and dresses the officer's head with a bandage. Outcomes are usually poor owing primarily to the underlying injury but also to the likely onset of brain infection.

In modern neurosurgical practice, there is a procedure called cutting burr holes in the skull, akin to trephining. It is used to relieve brain pressure after trauma from blood or fluid or to obtain a brain biopsy.

Stabbing and Cutting Wounds

From bayonets or swords, stabbing and cutting wounds were common but varied. The treatment depended upon their location, depth, and appearance. As with gunshot wounds, most bayonet and sword wounds entering the chest or abdominal cavity were fatal, either immediately from hemorrhage or after a few days from pneumonia, peritonitis and shock. On the other hand, a superficial cutting or slashing wound was treated with closure by sutures of linen, silk, or cotton or by sticking plasters. The sutures were removed after a few days. Yet, even these more superficial wounds commonly became infected because of the lack of antiseptics and absence of sterile technique in closure. Deep, penetrating wounds of an extremity were dilated and bandaged but also likely became infected. If an abscess developed, it required drainage. If gangrene set in, an amputation was in order.

Cannonball Injuries

Injuries by round shot from field cannon caused great tissue destruction and usually death. For soldiers who made it to the regimental hospital, the surgeon's options were limited, mainly amputation for a shattered, torn off, or bleeding limb.

Fractures

With simple fractures of the limbs, the surgeon reduced the broken bones "as nearly as possible to their natural situation, and ... retain[ed] them there, by the most easy, simple, and effectual means".[1] Most commonly, this was performed by two assistants applying traction and counter-traction "with more or less violence ... until the extremities of the broken bone were brought opposite to each other when the Surgeon finishes the coaptation or setting".[2] Medications were applied to the set limb consisting of, for example, adhesive plasters or "the white of an egg with vinegar," and the limb was strapped in place by a splint or by specialized dressings such as the eighteen-tailed bandage.[3,4]

Eighteenth-Century surgeons treated complicated fractures by amputation. These complications included joint involvement, abscess or gangrene, shattered limbs, or severe bleeding. Treatment of compound fractures, in which the broken bone pierced the skin, was controversial. Practicing in large hospitals, some surgeons "of the most distinguished reputation" advised immediate amputation in almost every bad compound fracture because of the risk of deadly infection. Others working "in the country" argued against it. Jones speculated that surgeons in the large hospitals regularly saw lethal infections after compound fractures whereas country doctors rarely saw it[5].

---

[1] Jones, 31.

[2] Ibid.

[3] Jones, 38.

[4] Wilbur, 35.

[5] Jones, 45-46.

ANNOTATED MEDICAL AND MILITARY GLOSSARY

Acute intermittent porphyria - a rare, hereditary disorder of heme (a component of hemoglobin) metabolism. The disease causes a buildup of toxic compounds and causes a wide array of physical and mental symptoms. This diagnosis was widely accepted for King George III for nearly fifty years until effectively challenged in 2010.

"Brown Bess" - the nickname for the standard British infantry musket used during the Eighteenth Century. It was a smooth bore, flintlock weapon, affixed with a lock to mount a bayonet.

Canister shot - an artillery shot of a closed metal casing filled with small iron or lead shot, used against charging infantry.

Calomel - a mercury compound used for many purposes including treating syphilis and preparing for smallpox inoculation. Mercury compounds were very toxic.

Camp followers – women who were an unofficial part of the army. They cooked, sewed, and provided nursing-type care. Some engaged in prostitution. Camp followers were made up of wives, widows, or freed enslaved persons.

Carbine - a short-barreled musket used by dragoons and cavalry.

Cathartics - laxatives.

Cataplasm - see poultice.

Cellulitis - a spreading infection as of an arm or leg, characterized by redness, swelling, and pain. It was common after battle injuries or after surgery.

Chancre - a characteristic painless ulcer of early syphilis.

Chancroid - a sexually transmitted disease, characterized by a painful ulcer, now rare in the United States. It is caused by the microorganism *Haemophilus ducreyi*.

Child mortality - the death rate between birth and age five years.

Chlamydia - the most common sexually transmitted (venereal) infection in the United States. It causes penile discharge in men and lower genital discharge and salpingitis in women. The infecting microorganism is *Chlamydia trachomatis*.

Cholecystitis - inflammation or infection of the gall bladder, possible diagnosis for General Nathaneal Greene in 1775-1776.

"Clap," the - a term for still used today for gonorrhea. Its origin may arise from the French term for brothels, les clapiers.

Cowpox - a mild skin infection caused by the cowpox virus which is related to the deadly smallpox virus. In 1796, Dr. Edward Jenner in England developed the first vaccine against smallpox by using material from a woman with cowpox of her hand.

Dragoons - mounted infantry.

Dura mater - the membranous lining of the brain and spinal cord.

Emaciation - marked thinness and weakness, usually from disease or starvation

Emetics - medication to cause vomiting

Endocarditis - infection of the heart valves, a complication of several infections including gonorrhea.

Epidemiology - the medical discipline dealing with occurrence and control of diseases.

Epiglottitis - infection or inflammation of the upper airway, likely the fatal diagnosis for George Washington in December 1799.

Flanking march - opposite of a direct frontal assault, a circuitous march to attack from the enemy's side. Used by British at the Battle of Long Island and at the Battle of the Brandywine.

Fomites – an inanimate item such as a blanket or clothing which can be contaminated with and spread a disease such as smallpox.

Gout- a disease caused by buildup of uric acid crystals in joints, the urinary tract, and other organs. With its hallmark findings of exquisitely painful inflammation of usually one (but sometimes more) joint, notably of the great toe, gout has been recognized since ancient times. Because it has been long associated with rich foods and excessive alcohol, gout has been referred to as "the disease of kings." It affected Benjamin Franklin, American General Charles Lee, British statesman William Pitt, and many others.

Grape shot- an artillery shot of a tightly packed canvas bag filled with small iron or lead shot, used against charging infantry.

Gumma – a manifestation of syphilis, a hard, raised tumor-like bump.

Hepatitis - infection or inflammation of the liver, a possible diagnosis for General Nathaneal Greene in 1775-1776.

Humors - The Eighteenth-Century principles of medicine maintained that the body fluids or "humors" needed to be in balance for health. The four humors and their associated features were identified as blood, phlegm, yellow bile, and black bile. Conversely, it was believed that an imbalance of the humors caused disease. It was therefore internally consistent that, to treat disease, balance of the humors had to be restored. Accordingly, physicians practiced bloodletting and leech applications to remove an excess of blood, emetics to induce vomiting, or cathartics to expel excessive bowel fluid.

Lancet - a sharp instrument for letting blood, also called a fleam.

Lazaretto – a pest house.

Ligating – tying off, as a bleeding blood vessel.

Mate, Surgeon's- a surgeon's assistant.

Macule – small reddish spots.

Miasmata - unhealthy smells or vapors as from marshy or swampy ground, thought to be the cause of malaria in the Eighteenth Century.

Midwifery – the practice of obstetrics, care of pregnant women, especially the delivery of the infant.

Mortar - a type of artillery with a high arched, lobbing trajectory.

Necrotizing-causing necrosis, death of body tissue, as in a severe infection.

Offal - the internal organs of a butchered animal.

Papule - a small, red, raised bump.

Paroxysm - an attack of a disease such as malaria.

Parasiticide – a medication for a parasitic infection such as malaria.

Pericarditis - infection or inflammation of the sac lining the heart. It is a complication of several infections including disseminated gonorrhea.

Peritonitis - infection or inflammation of the lining of the abdominal cavity. It complicated wounds of the abdomen was fatal in the Eighteenth Century.

Petechiae - small red spots caused by bleeding into the skin.

Pharyngitis - infection of the upper airway.

Phlebotomy - removal of blood from a vein, as in bloodletting or drawing blood for a test.

Plasters - adhesive bandages.

Poultice - a moist soothing dressing, also called a cataplasm.

Proctitis - infection of the rectum. It may be a complication of gonorrhea.

Purgative - a laxative.

Quinsy - a severe throat infection.

Salpingitis - infection of the fallopian tubes which lead from the ovary to the uterus, caused by gonorrhea, chlamydia and other microorganisms. It causes pain and sterility and may lead to a tubal pregnancy.

Scabies - an itching skin infestation caused by mites, burrowing insects.

Septicemia - blood poisoning, a type of life-threatening infection.

Siege - a tactic used against a well-fortified position, blocking food, supplies and reinforcements.

Spicules - sharp, pointed fragments as of bone.

Suppuration - formation and discharge of pus.

Tenesmus - a constant feeling of needing to move one's bowels.

Thoracentesis - placing a needle into the chest cavity to remove blood, pus, trapped air, or fluid.

Tincture - a medication dissolved in alcohol.

Trephining - removal of a disc of skull bone to decrease pressure on the brain as after trauma or a wound.

Typhus - an infection spread by the human body louse, usually in crowded conditions such as in wartime or refugee camps. It was characterized by fever and a petechial rash. With a high mortality, typhus was called ship, jail, camp or hospital fever in the Eighteenth Century.

Ureter - tubular structure leading from kidney to bladder.

Urethra - the tubular structure exiting the bladder. In males, it passes the length of the penis.

Vector - an organism that spreads disease from one person or animal to another, as mosquitoes in malaria and the body louse in typhus.

Venesection - opening of a vein, phlebotomy.

Vesicles - small, fluid filled blisters, as in early smallpox or in herpes infection.

NOTES ON REFERENCES

Based on a lifetime of reading and studying medicine, I wrote *1776, Medicine* and *War* as a tour of the medical landscape in Eighteenth-Century North America. Throughout the book, I have aimed to put knowledge and practice of that era in the context of modern medicine. Overall, my references span 300 years. For generally known facts such as the course of the war or common medical knowledge, I have not given specific references. For any key sources that I missed citing, I offer my sincere apologies.

I have categorized the references as: primary sources including original records, journals and memoirs; books written well after the war; and articles mainly from scholarly journals. To fill in gaps, I turned to sources on the internet. I tried to rely upon credible websites, but I acknowledge problems with these sources. Websites are not peer-reviewed, and sites change, come and go.

Primary Sources

Bauremeister, CL. *Revolution in America: Confidential Letters and Journal 1776-1784*. (B A Uhlendorf, Trans.). New Brunswick, NJ. 1957. (The author was a general commanding Hessian (German) forces as mercenaries for the British.)

Burgoyne, John. *Orderly book of Lt. General Burgoyne* (Notes by E B O'Callaghan). Albany, 1860.

Carleton Papers (Headquarters Papers of the British Army in America). 1968. Public Record Office, PRO 30/55, 107 vols. National Archives, Kew, UK. Accessed July 1968.

Digby, W. *Journal of Lt. William Digby* (James Phinney Baxter, Ed). Albany, 1889.

Hamilton, R. *The Duties of a Regimental Surgeon*, 2nd ed. London, 1794.

Hunter, John. *Observations on the Diseases of the Army in Jamaica*. London,1788. (Author is a different John Hunter from the famed Eighteenth-Century English surgeon.)

Jones, John. *Plain Concise Practical Remarks, on the Treatment of Wounds and Fractures*. Philadelphia, Robert Bell Publisher,1776.

Osler, W. *The Principles and Practice of Medicine*, fifth edition. New York, D. Appleton & Co, 1903. (Written decades before the antibiotic era by a medical giant of the time, the text provides vivid, detailed pictures of disease as they would have been seen in the late 18th Century. I used my tattered, personal copy.)

Riedesel, FA. *Memories of Major General Riedesel* (Max von Eelking, Trans and Wm. L Stone, Ed). Albany, 1868. (The author was another German commanding officer.)

Rollo, John. *Observations of Diseases which Appeared in the Army on St. Lucia in 1778 and 1779* (London) 1781.

Royal Comm. On Hist. Manuscripts, 1910: 36, *Arbuthnot to Germain, 25 August 1779* (accessed July 1968).

Rush, Benjamin. *Directions For Preserving The Health of Soldiers*. Philadelphia,1777.

Senter, Isaac. *The Journal of Isaac Senter. Physician and Surgeon to the Troops Detached from the American Army Encamped at Cambridge, Mass, on a Secret Expedition Against Quebec, under the Command of Col. Benedict Armold, in September 1775*. Philadelphia: Published by the Historical Society of Pennsylvania, 1846. Tarrytown, New York, Reprinted William Abbatt, 1915.

Tilton, James, *Economical Observations on Military Hospitals and Prevention and Cure of Diseases Incident to an Army*. Wilmington Del, 1813.

War Office. *17 Monthly Returns 1759–1865*. Vol. 17, *1776–1782*. n.p., n.d. Accessed July 1968.

Books

Abrams, Jeanne. *Revolutionary Medicine, The Founding Fathers and Mothers in Sickness and Health. New York.* New York University Press, 2013.

Alden, John Richard. *General Charles Lee, Traitor or Patriot?* Baton Rouge, Louisiana State University Press,1951.

Atkinson Rick. *The British Are Coming, The War for America, Lexington to Princeton, 1775-1777*, Volume One of *The Revolution Trilogy*, New York, Henry Holt, 2019.

Atkinson Rick. *The Fate of the Day, The War for America, Fort Ticonderoga to Charleston, 1777-1780*, Volume Two of *The Revolution Trilogy*, New York, Crown, 2025.

Blake J.B. *Public Health in the Town of Boston 1630-1822*. Cambridge, Harvard Univ Press, 1959.

Cantlie N. *A History of the Army Medical Department, Vol I*, Edinburgh and London, Churchill and Livingstone, 1974.

Curtis Edward E. *The Organization of the British Army in the American Revolution*. London, 1929.

Duncan L.C. *Medical men in the American Revolution (1775-1783.)* New York, Augustus M Kelley, Publishers,1971. (First Published by Medical Field Service School, Carlisle Barracks, 1931).

di Spigna, Christian. *Founding Martyr, The Life and Death of Dr. Joseph Warren, The American Revolution's Lost Hero*. New York, Crown, 2018.

Freeman, Douglas Southall, *Washington, An Abridgement in one volume* by Richard Harwell of the seven volume George Washington. New York, Charles Scribner's Sons,1968.

Fried, S. Rush: Revolution, *Madness and the Visionary Doctor who Became a Founding Father*. New York, Crown, 2019

Gibson J.E. *Dr. Bodo Otto and the Medical Background of the American Revolution*, Springfield, Ill, Charles C. Thomas, 1937

Gifford. G. *Physician Signers of the Declaration of Independence*. New York, Science History Publications, a division of Neale Watson Academic Publications, Inc, 1976. (This book, published over fifty years ago, provided excellent background and insight about prominent early American physician-statesmen.)

Longo D, Fauci A, Kasper D et al. *Harrison's Principles of Internal Medicine, 22nd edition*, New York, McGraw Hill, 2026. This is an authoritative current text of internal medicine.

Hasselgren P-O. *Revolutionary Surgeons, Patriots and Loyalists on the Cutting Edge*, New York, Knox Press, 2021.

Larson EJ. *Franklin and Washington*. New York, Harper Collins, 2020.

Millard C. *Destiny of the Republic: A Tale of Murder of a President*. New York, Doubleday, 2011.

Philbrick N. *Valiant Ambition, George Washington, Benedict Arnold, and the Fate of the Revolution*. New York, Viking, 2016.

Reiss O. *Medicine and The American Revolution, How Diseases and Their Treatments Affected the Colonial Army*. Jefferson, NC, McFarland & Co, Jefferson, 1998.

Roberts A. *The Last King of America, The Misunderstood Reign of George III*. New York, Viking, 2021.

Stanley G. *For Want of a Horse*. Sackville, NB, 1961.

Wehrman AM. *The Contagion of Liberty, The Politics of Smallpox in the American Revolution*. Baltimore, Johns Hopkins University Press, 2022.

Wilbur CK. *Revolutionary Medicine 1700-1800*, Second Edition. Guilford CT, Globe Press, 1997.

Wildes HE. *Valley Forge*, MacMillan Company, New York, 1938.

Articles, including on-line journals

Chang CY, Goldstein E, Agarwal N et al. "Ether in the developing world: rethinking an abandoned agent." *BMC Anesthesiology*. 2015;15:149.

Dunea G. "William Pitt: Father and Son," *Hektoen International, A Journal of Medical Humanities*, hekint.org (accessed December 11, 2025).

Editorial. "Sir John Pringle (1707-1782)—Military Physician and Hygienist." *Journal of the American Medical Association*, 190: 113-14, 1964.

Gensel, Lisa. "The Medical World of Benjamin Franklin." *Journal of the Royal Society of Medicine* 98, no. 12 (December 2005): 534–38.

Griesemer, Abigail D., William D. Widmann, Kenneth A. Forde, and Mark A. Hardy. "John Jones, MD: Pioneer, Patriot, and Founder of American Surgery." *World Journal of Surgery* 34, no. 4 (April 2010): 605–609.

Griffenhagen G. "Drug Supplies in the American Revolution," *United States National Museum Bulletin* 225, Smithsonian Institution,1961.

Hasselgren, Per-Olaf. 2020. "The Smallpox Epidemics in America in the 1700s and the Role of the Surgeons: Lessons to be Learned During the Global Outbreak of COVID-19." *World Journal of Surgery* 44, no. 9 (September 2020): 2837–41.

Jones DS, Podolsky SH, Barr J. "Smallpox at the Siege of Boston, November 1775-March 1776," *New England Journal of Medicine* 2025; 393: 2281-84.

Jose, P. P., et al. "Gonorrhea: Historical Outlook." *Journal of Skin and Sexually Transmitted Diseases* 2, no. 2 (2020): 110–14.

Katz A. "That 'Terrible' 1777 Valley Forge Winter Called Just Average." *The Evening Bulletin*, December 22, 1965.

MacAlpine I, Hunter R. "The Insanity of King George III, a Classic Case of Porphyria," *British Medical Journal*, 8 January 1966; 65-71.

McGready Blake. "Abigail Hartman Rice, Revolutionary War Nurse". *Journal of the American Revolution* November 28, 2016, allthingsliberty.com/2016/11/ abigail-hartman-rice-revolutionary-war-nurse/.

Mikhael M and Siva C, "Dialogue Between Franklin and the Gout Reexamined," *Clinical Medicine and Research* 2023; 21(4):196-200).

Montressor, John. "Journals of Captain John Montressor." In *Collections of the New-York Historical Society for the Year 1881*. Vol. 14. New York: Printed for the Society, 1882.

Morens DM. "Death of a President." *New England Journal of Medicine* 1999;341; 1845-49.

Parascandola J. "Drug Therapy in Colonial and Revolutionary America," *American Journal of Hospital Pharmacy* (later renamed to the *American Journal of Health-System Pharmacy*). 1976; 33:807-10.

Peters TJ, Wilkinson D. "King George III and Porphyria: a clinical re-examination of the historical evidence," *History of Psychiatry*, 2010, 21(10:3-19.).

Pinals, Robert S. "How Admiral Rodney's disability saved the American Revolution." *The Pharos*, Spring 2021.

Rosenberg, Chaim M. "Early Medical Education and the Revolutionary War", *Journal of The American Revolution*, April 15, 2025.

Shanks GD. "Malaria Influenced Outcomes of Yorktown Sieges:1781 and 1862," *American Journal of Tropical Medicine and Hygiene* 113 (2), 2025, 278-281.

Sheldon GF. "The Westward Expansion and Surgical Practice in America." *Bulletin of the America College of Surgeons* 1998; 83: 10-24.

Tampa M, Sarbu I , Matel et al. "Brief History of Syphilis," *Journal Medicine and Life* 2014; Mar 25;7(1) 4-10.

Thursfield, Hugh. "Smallpox in the American War of Independence." *Annals of Medical History*, 3rd ser., 2, no. 4 (July 1940): 312–18.

Thoms H. "Albigence Waldo, Surgeon, His Diary Written at Valley Forge," *Annals of Medical History*. 10:486, 1928.

Turley, John. "250th Series: Medicine in the Time of the Revolution." *SAR Magazine* 115, no. 2 (Fall 2020). Massachusetts Society, Sons of the American Revolution. https://massar.org/250th-series-medicine-in-the-time-of-the-revolution/.

Waring JI. "Medicine in Charleston at the Time of the Revolution," *Journal of the American Medical Association* 236; 31-34, 1976.

Wilkinson, Lise, "'The Other' John Hunter, MD (1754-1809): His Contributions to The Medical Literature, and To The Introduction of Animal Experiments into Infectious Disease Research". *Notes and Records of the Royal Society of London*, Feb 1982, Vol 36, No, 2. Pp 227-241.

Websites

AMEDD Center of History & Heritage, “Surgeons General: Benjamin Church,” achh.army.mil/history/surgeongenerals-b-church, website accessed March 2, 2026.

AMEDD Center of History & Heritage , “Surgeons General: J. Tilton,” achh.army.mil/history/surgeongenerals-j-tilton, website accessed March 2, 2026.

American Battlefield Trust. 2020. “Healing Heroines.” Head-Tilting History. March 19, 2020. Accessed February 16, 2026. https://www.battlefields.org/learn/head-tilting-history/healing-heroines.

American Battlefield Trust. “Hugh Mercer.” Accessed December 18, 2025. battlefields.org.

American Revolutionary War Continental Regiments, accessed Feb 6, 2026 revolutionarywar.us/continental-army/massachusetts,

American Revolution Facts, Updated October 14, 2025, www.battlefields.org/learn/articles/american-revolution-faqs, accessed December 17, 2025.

Army Medicine Facebook Post, May 6, 2025. Nurses During the Revolutionary War, accessed February 16, 2026.

B2B Staffing Services. "The Unsung Patriots: How Nursing Helped Win the Revolutionary War." July 3, 2025. b2bstaffingservices.com/nursing-helped-win-the-revolutionary-war, accessed February 16, 2026.

Crossroads of the American Revolution. “Hugh Mercer Full Biography,” accessed December 18, 2025. https://revolutionarynj.org/people_biography/hugh-mercer-full-biography/.

Dental Care in Early America. Lives and legaciesblog.org/2015/09/02/dental-care-in-early-America, accessed Aug 8, 2025; loomisroaddental.com/colonial-dental-treatments.

Dr. Bodo Otto Association , www.drbodootto.org/biography, accessed February 26, 2026.

Ellis, Marietta and Arthur. “Colonial Soap Making—Its History and Techniques,” accessed December 13, 2025. www.garuolds.com>files>Colonial Soap.

Centers for Disease Control. “Fast stats—Life expectancy,” www.cdc.gov>nchs>fastats, accessed December 13, 2025.

Fort Greene Park Monuments-Prison Ship Martyrs www.nycgovparks.org>parks>monuments, accessed September 22, 2025.

Greenwalt, Philip. “Soldier Pay in the American Revolution” American Battlefield Trust, Updated December 18, 2023. www.battlefields.org, accessed April 6, 2026.

History of Pennsylvania Hospital, uphs.upenn.edu, accessed September 18, 2025.

Kraemer, Matthew. “American Suffering Aboard the HMS Jersey, New Jersey as a Battleground”, www.revnj.org/blog/hms-jersey. accessed September 20, 2025.

Monmouth Battle Facts and Summary/ American Battlefield Trust, accessed February 20, 2026, www.battlefields.org/learn/revolutionary-war/monmouth.

Najera Rene F, “Washington’s War Against Smallpox: The Revolutionary Inoculation Campaign.” April 7, 2025. historyofvacines.org/blog/washingtons-war-against-smallpox-revolutionary-inoculation-campaign, accessed January 24, 2026.

Ingraham, Courtland D. McE. “Philip John Schuyler” George Washington’s Mount Vernon, Digital Encyclopedia, accessed April 6, 2026, www.mountvernon.org/library/digitalhistory/digital-encyclopedia/article/philip-john-schuyler-1733-1804.

Jenrich, Charles H. "The Old Jersey Prison Ship." Proceedings, February 1963. www.usni.org>proceedings>february>old-jersey accessed September 21, 2025.

Price, David. “Albigence Waldo: Surgeon, Soldier, Diarist, Poet”, *Washington Crossing Historic Park*, www.washingtoncrossingpark.org/albigence-waldo-surgeon-soldier-diarist-poet, accessed, January 17, 2026.

Salotto, Lori, comp. 2000. "Dr. Isaac Senter Papers." Rhode Island Historical Society, Manuscripts Division. Accessed January 17, 2026. rihs.org.

"Smallpox, Inoculation, and the Revolutionary War". www.nps.gov/articles/000/smallpox-inoculation-revolutionary-war.htm, accessed January 20, 2026.

"Surgery in the 1700s" www.encyclopedia.com/science/encyclopedias-almanacs-transcripts-and-maps/surgery-1700s, accessed July 28, 2025.

"The physical challenges of Major General Nathaneal Greene". battleofrhodeisland.org/the-physical-challenges-of-major-general-nathaneal-greene, accessed December 9, 2025.

"The 9 Deadly Diseases That Plagued George Washington", PBS News, July 4, 2011 www.pbs.org/newshour/health/george-washingtons-medical-chart accessed December 7, 2025.

To Bathe or Not to Bathe. Coming Clean in Colonial America by Edwards Park., research.colonialwillamsburg.org/foundation/journ, accessed December 18, 2025.

U S Army Revolutionary War 250th Commemoration 2025-2033) The Fighting Man of the Continental Army, Daily Life as a Soldier, Updated July 26, 2024). (www.battlefields.org/learn/articles/fighting-man-continental-army accessed December 19, 2025.

Uva, Katie. "Benedict Arnold", *George Washington's Mount Vernon Digital Encyclopedia*, www.mountvernon.org/library/digitalhistory/digital-encyclopedia/article/benedict-arnold, accessed December 18, 2025.

Valley Forge, 1777-1778. "Diary of Surgeon Albigence Waldo, of the Connecticut Line (Full Text)", archive.org/stream/jstor-20085750/20085750_djvu.txt. Accessed January 17, 2026.

Washington Papers, washingtonpapers.org/resources/articles/supply-problems-plagued-the-continental-army-from-the-start. Accessed August 8, 2025.

Whelan, Jean C. n.d. "American Nursing: An Introduction to the Past." *Nursing, History, and Health Care*. University of Pennsylvania School of Nursing. www.nursing.upenn.edu/nhhc/american-nursing-an-introduction-to-the-past/. Accessed February 16, 2016.

Wikipedia contributors, "John Hunter (physician)," *Wikipedia, The Free Encyclopedia*, en.wikipedia.org/w/index.php?title=John_Hunter_(physician)&oldid=1332139433, accessed December 18, 2025).

www.ingramcontent.com/pod-product-compliance
Lightning Source LLC
LaVergne TN
LVHW022211200926
848481LV00006B/1928
9798996770502